Hemoperfusion

Contributions to Nephrology

Vol. 29

S. Karger · Basel · München · Paris · London · New York · Sydney

International Meeting on Hemoperfusion, Bologna, March 16, 1981

Hemoperfusion

Volume Editors
V. Bonomini, Bologna and *T.M.S. Chang,* Montreal

45 figures and 55 tables, 1982

S. Karger · Basel · München · Paris · London · New York · Sydney

Contributions to Nephrology

National Library of Medicine, Cataloging in Publication
International Meeting on Hemoperfusion
(1981: Bologna, Italy)
Hemoperfusion
International Meeting on Hemoperfusion, Bologna, March 16, 1981;
volume editors, V. Bonomini and T.M.S. Chang.
Basel; New York: Karger, 1982.
(Contributions to Nephrology; v. 29)
1. Hemoperfusion - congress I. Bonomini V.
II. Chang, Thomas Ming Swi III. Title
IV. Series
WI CO778UN v. 29
[WG 168 1595h 1981]
ISBN 3-8055-3421-3

Drug Dosage

The author and publisher have exerted every effort to ensure that drug selection and dosage set forth in this text are in accord with current recommendations and practice at the time of publication. However, in view of ongoing research, changes in government regulations, and the constant flow of information relating to drug therapy and drug reactions, the reader is urged to check the package insert for each drug for any change in indications and dosage and for added warnings and precautions. This is particularly important when the recommended agent is a new and/or infrequently employed drug.

Satz: Satzstudio Frohberg, D-6463 Freigericht
Printed in Switzerland by Thür AG Offsetdruck, Pratteln
ISBN 3-8055-3421-3

Contents

Welcoming Address

As chairman of the local organizing committee I would like to thank all the distinguished speakers who agreed to participate in this 'International Meeting on Hemoperfusion'. We were proud to welcome to Bologna the leading investigators of the world in this most sophisticated interdisciplinary field of clinical research, hemoperfusion, where nephrology joins hands with toxicology, pharmacology, bioengineering, immunology and other fields of medicine. I am sure we will benefit greatly by the papers presented.

The 'International Meeting on Hemoperfusion' forms part of a teaching and research program that the Postgraduate School of Nephrology of the University of Bologna periodically devotes to enhancement in clinical nephrology.

The first title of the workshop was to have been 'Charcoal Hemoperfusion in Chronic Uremia'. It was expanded to 'Hemoperfusion' both because other systems of perfusion besides activated charcoal are currently employed (resins above all), and because hemoperfusion has found application in other fields besides uremia: some well-established, such as poisoning and liver failure, others here to be disclosed for the first time, like diabetic coma. The updated title 'International Meeting on Hemoperfusion' does justice to the range and topicality of our speakers' investigations, and I should once more like to thank them for accepting our invitation.

My special thanks go to Prof. *G.E. Schreiner,* President of the International Society of Nephrology, Prof. *C. Rizzoli,* Rector of the University of Bologna, and Prof. *M. Zanetti,* Director of the St. Orsola University Hospital, who all honored the meeting with their presence. My deepest personal gratitude to Prof. *T.M.S. Chang,* who most kindly consented to act as editor of this volume, together with myself. I am also indebted to the series editors, Prof. *G. Berlyne* and *S. Giovannetti,* for their goodwill and friendly cooperation in agreeing to publish the congress material. Lastly, I should convey our appreciation to the publishers themselves for their customary efficiency and accuracy in bringing out the proceedings of our meeting.

Vittorio Bonomini, Bologna

Contr. Nephrol., vol. 29, pp. 1–2 (Karger, Basel 1982)

Foreword on Hemoperfusion and Uremia

V. Bonomini

Department of Nephrology and Dialysis, St. Orsola University Hospital, Bologna, Italy

It is a well-known fact that the use of hemoperfusion involves various fields of medicine. In some of them (hepatic failure, acute intoxication) its application is sporadic, while in others hemoperfusion procedures have to be repeated cyclically and regularly over a long period. This is the case with hemoperfusion in patients affected by chronic renal failure [2]. Such treatment involves various aspects, clinical, ethical, social as well as economic, many of which are still to be clarified.

Regular hemodialysis treatment affords long-term survival of patients affected by chronic renal failure. To date, the kidney is the only internal organ in the whole area of medicine whose abolished function is replaced effectively, totally and over long periods of time, by an organ artificially made by man's technology. Thousands of people are at present treated with artificial kidneys all over the world.

The need to clarify the role of hemoperfusion in chronic dialysis points to a certain dissatisfaction with the clinical results afforded by technology. Certainly, if we could hold a championship of internal artificial organs, the artificial kidney would walk off with the gold medal: without dialysis, indeed, life would not be possible. It is similarly certain, however, that the gold medal has another side: most uremic changes, in fact, persist in survivors. Technically adequate dialysis, therefore, does not always coincide with clinically adequate results, and we should not confuse the dialysis capacity to rehabilitate the patient for working with the dialysis incapacity to rehabilitate the patient from uremia.

In spite of the hundreds of papers on this topic leading to a sort of pollution in words and ideas, we do not know exactly why this occurs, the two possible alternatives being mere conjectures: (1) the effect of losing the incretory along with the excretory renal function, and (2) a still inadequate removal of toxins because of their size and bonds.

At least two clinical facts support the validity of the first point: (1) effective clinical rehabilitation from advanced uremia is only achievable by renal transplantation; (2) the possible prevention of advancing uremia by early dialysis

[1] where renal and extrarenal endocrine levels are still satisfactorily preserved. However, since dialysis tends to be started late for a wide spectrum of reasons (from prejudice to inevitability) and most uremic problems are not reversed, some new technological areas should be explored in the hope of enhancing present clinical results.

The use of sorbents (above all charcoal) in uremic patients has to be regarded in this light as a potential technical approach to ameliorate artificial substitution therapy. Owing to its wide spectrum in adsorptive capacity, but also its intrinsic limits (poor biocompatibility, inability to remove urea, electrolytes and water, and cost), charcoal hemoperfusion can at present be regarded only as a valid adjunct rather than an alternative to hemodialysis treatment.

Increased biocompatibility has been achieved in recent years by coating the charcoal granules with various highly reliable coating membranes [*Chang,* this volume]. This allows a safer and wider use of charcoal in chronic uremia and the fullest exploitation of its adsorptive capacity: substances of the middle molecular range are removed as well as small molecules. It is still unclear what role, if any, the so-called middle molecules play in determining the uremic syndrome. However, the intrinsic capacity of charcoal for removing many such molecules together with positive results achieved by several authors using hemoperfusion are points of undeniable interest.

As for our own experience with charcoal, it falls into three phases: oral administration (20 years ago), insertion in the dialysis circuit (15 years ago) and, most recently, direct insertion in the blood circuit. The first two phases yielded quite unsatisfactory results; the third proves encouraging in terms of patients' clinical improvement and/or time saved. The two goals are of primary importance as far as longterm treatment of chronic uremic patients is concerned.

The basic assumptions of our study together with characteristics of patients, general schedules of treatment and results are reported in detail [*Stefoni* et al., this volume]. It seems to us that, though advantages are mixed with drawbacks as with all other technology, the appropriate use of charcoal hemoperfusion does make a valuable contribution in improving the results of artificial substitution therapy of chronic renal failure.

References

1 Bonomini, V.: Early dialysis 1979. Nephron *24:* 157 (1979).
2 Winchester, J.F.; Gelfand, M.C.; Knepshield, J.H.; Schreiner, G.E.: Present and future uses of hemoperfusion with sorbents. Int. J. artif. Organs *2:* 353 (1978).

V. Bonomini, MD, Department of Nephrology and Dialysis,
St. Orsola University Hospital, I–40100 Bologna (Italy)

Contr. Nephrol., vol. 29, pp. 3–6 (Karger, Basel 1982)

Forward on Hemoperfusion and Artificial Cells

T.M.S. Chang

Artificial Cells and Organs Research Centre, McGill University, Montreal, Quebec, Canada

Progress in biomedical sciences follows interesting routes. In many cases it requires research from many initially unrelated areas to arrive at practical therapeutic approaches. The field of clinical applications of hemoperfusion is one example of this.

As early as 1948, *Muirhead and Reid* [4] had studied the possible use of resin hemoperfusion in animal study and as early as 1958 *Schreiner* [6] had tested this clinically. However, because of the problem of blood incompatibility this has not received wide acceptance despite continued research especially by *Rosenbaum* et al. [5] to improve this system. In the case of charcoal hemoperfusion, *Yatzidis* [7] has carried out clinical trials as early as 1964. However, the problem of platelet depletion and charcoal embolism had resulted in the discontinuation of uncoated charcoal hemoperfusion in patients shortly after that time.

Work has been carried out since 1957 by *Chang* [1] on a completely unrelated area of artificial cells. This had in 1966 [2] resulted in the demonstration that the principle of artificial cells can be used for microencapsulation of enzymes, charcoal (fig. 1) and resins (fig. 2) for use in hemoperfusion. Furthermore, it was also demonstrated here that albumin coating could be used to make the surface completely blood-compatible for hemoperfusion (albumin-collodion activated charcoal, ACAC) [3]. The demonstration here of the safety and applications of the hemoperfusion system [3] in uremia, acute intoxication and hepatic coma has resulted in considerable interest in the clinical application of charcoal hemoperfusion. More recently this interest has also been extended to the use of the principle of artificial cells for resin hemoperfusion in which either the microencapsulation technique or the albumin coating technique has been applied to resin hemoperfusion. Further extension also includes the use of im-

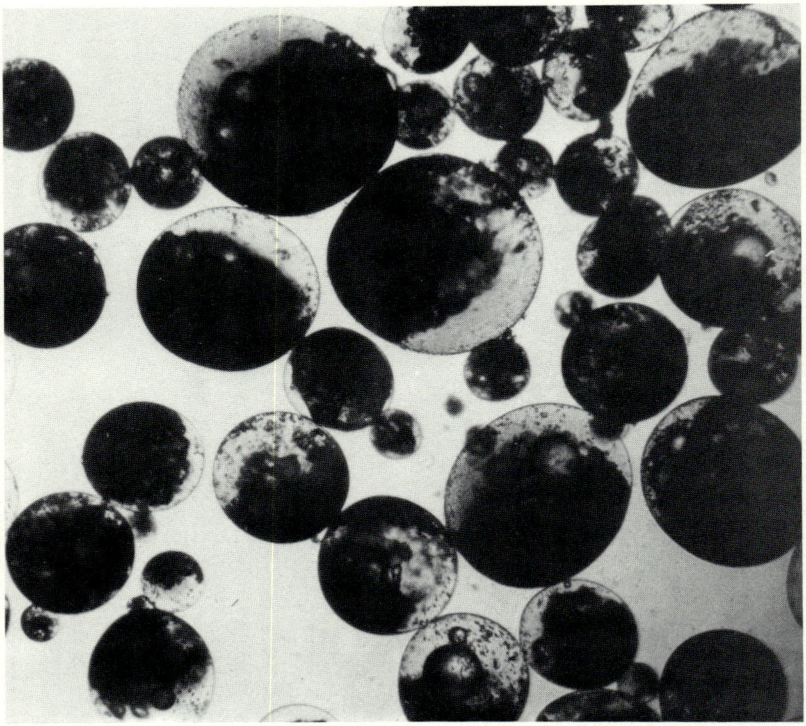

Fig. 1. One type of microencapsulated activated charcoal used in 1966 for hemoperfusion [2].

mobilized enzymes, blood-compatible immunoadsorbent, and other systems for use in hemoperfusion. Other approaches are also being developed to avoid the need for artificial cells in hemoperfusion. For instance, some centers are now working on charcoal particles which are strong enough so as not to cause embolism even without membrane coating, but blood compatibility may still be a problem. Perhaps albumin coating will help. In any case, we should all keep an open mind to develop the best hemoperfusion system irrespective of the final approach.

Extensive clinical trials and large-scale assessment will only be possible with the availability of large-scale industrial production. Effectiveness has been rightfully sacrificed for safety in the earlier stages of industrial development. With further experience gained in industrial production improved systems are being

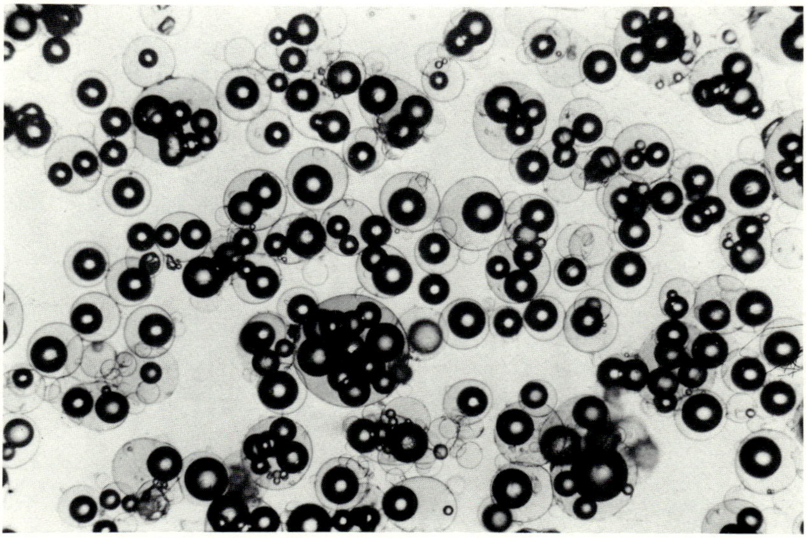

Fig. 2. Microencapsulation of resins used in hemoperfusion in 1966 [2].

produced by many companies and some of the systems are approaching the laboratory-produced ACAC system in efficiency and blood compatibility. At this stage of development of hemoperfusion it will be most important to use only the best industrially produced hemoperfusion system. Otherwise, the clinical and laboratory results obtained will be confusing. Many centers have had such bad experiences from commercial hemoperfusion systems of low efficiency and low blood compatibility that they are now great opponents of hemoperfusion.

It is gratifying to see from this symposium that many commercially produced hemoperfusion systems are continuing to be improved. May I make a plea to all industries to continue this good work of improving their systems and to discard those which are not as effective or as blood-compatible. With any new therapeutic method, the medical profession rightfully wants to be particularly careful in assessing any new approaches before they are used routinely in patients. This can only be done by carefully assessing the clinical applications of hemoperfusion in different conditions using valid scientific data obtained with good hemoperfusion systems. To this end, the present symposium is an excellent opportunity for discussing and comparing results obtained by different groups around the world.

References

1 Chang, T.M.S.: Semipermeable microcapsules. Science *146:* 524–524 (1964).
2 Chang, T.M.S.: Semipermeable aqueous microcapsules ('artificial cells'): with emphasis on experiments in an extracorporeal shunt system. Trans. Am. Soc. artif. internal Organs *12:* 13–19 (1966).
3 Chang, T.M.S.: Removal of endogenous and exogenous toxins by a microencapsulated absorbent. Can. J. Physiol. Pharmacol. *47:* 1043–1045 (1969).
4 Muirhead, E.E.; Reid, A.F.: A resin artificial kidney. J. Lab. clin. Med. *33:* 841–844 (1948).
5 Rosenbaum, J.; Kramer, M.S.; Raja, R.; Boreyko, C.: Resin hemoperfusion. New Engl. J. Med. *284:* 874–877 (1971).
6 Schreiner, G.E.: The role of hemodialysis in acute poisoning. Archs intern. Med. *102:* 896–900 (1958).
7 Yatzidis, H.: A convenient hemoperfusion micro-apparatus over charcoal for the treatment of endogenous and exogenous intoxications. Proc. Eur. Dial. Trans. Ass. *1:* 83–87 (1964).

Prof. T.M.S. Chang, Artificial Cells and Organs Research Centre, McGill University, H3G 1Y6 Montreal, Quebec (Canada)

Contr. Nephrol., vol. 29, pp. 7–10 (Karger, Basel 1982)

Clinical Hemoperfusion

George E. Schreiner

Georgetown University Medical Center, Washington, D.C., USA

The blood stream is the macrotransport system of biology, through which everything we inhale, ingest or inject is transported. Biologically effective molecules such as nutrients, drugs and toxic chemical are either transported in free solution, bound to specific proteins (e.g. ceruloplasmin), bound to general plasma proteins (e.g. albumin), or bound to cells. From this macrotransport system, biologically active cells receive molecules either by (a) diffusion along a concentration gradient: intravascular → extracellular → cellular, or (b) specific receptors which compete against whatever binding energy exists between target molecules and the transport protein in the serum or the receptor site on the cell membrane.

All binding energies are relative. If one dips a strip of cellophane into an aqueous or saline solution of the dye T-1824 (Evans blue dye), the cellophane will come up blue (i.e. the cellophane can bind to the dye). But if one adds albumin to the solution first, then dips the cellophane, it comes up clear. Thus, binding energy of the albumin for T-1824 is greater than that of the cellophane. Further, if one injects T-1824 albumin into an animal or a man with a large amyloid liver, the liver will turn blue. Thus, the binding energy of amyloid for T-1824 is greater than that of albumin. This simple experiment not only demonstrates the relativity of binding, but also gives us a practical warning signal as clinical investigators. It is critical that devices intended for ultimate use in a clinical setting be designed and tested using blood or plasma as a circulating medium even though it is a lot simpler and easier to carry out tests on aqueous or saline solutions.

These are the fundamental principles underlying clinical hemoperfusion, which is so beautifully delineated in this symposium. Essentially, hemoperfusion relies on general sorbents (e.g. activated charcoal) or specific sorbents (e.g. selected resins), with a high infinity for a selected target molecule. They are given physical characteristics (fine/coarse) to provide optimum surface area and mixing, and to meet such hemodynamic variables as pressure, flow and resistance. The sorbents are enclosed within a cartridge or chamber to maximize exchange. They

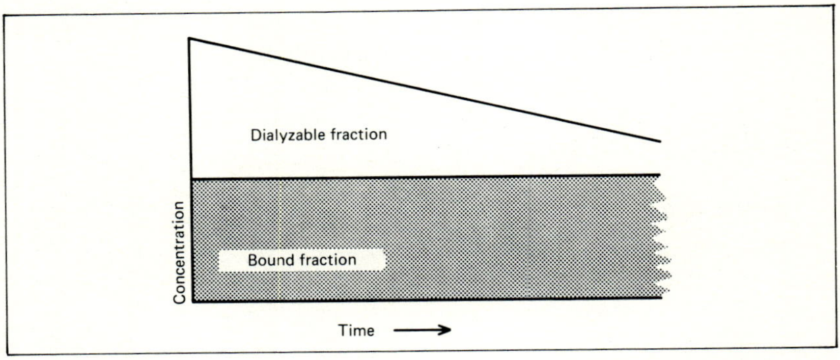

Fig. 1. Resin perfusion. Relationship of dialyzable to bound fraction of circulating solutes. Model shows progressive loss of dialyzable fraction with change in its relation to total blood level.

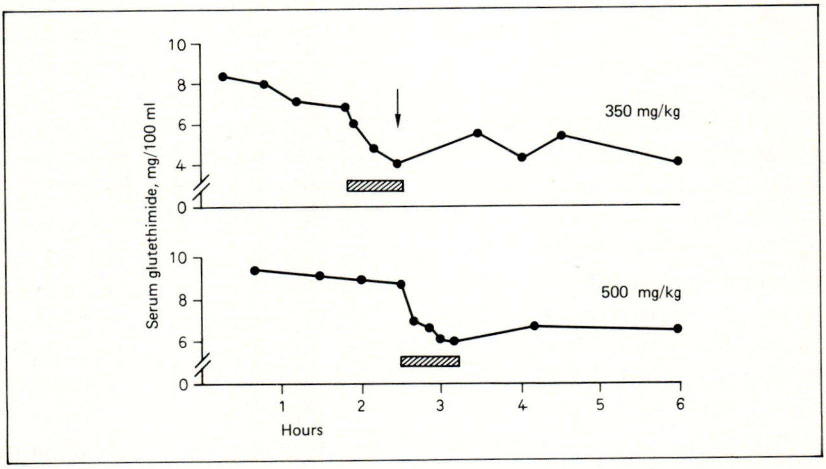

Fig. 2. Effect of short hemoperfusion on dogs with glutethimide intoxication.

are treated or coated to improve biocompatibility, the principal problem being circulating platelets. The most effective sorbent in terms of biocompatibility usually suffers from reduction in efficiency, and one must often trade off a fraction of efficacy for the necessary fraction of safety.

Optimism for reversal of tissue binding by depletion of plasma concentration was first afforded by the experiments of *Cutting and Koppanyi* [1] who infused saline into hitherto irreversibly comatose dogs with barbiturate overdose,

Table I. Criteria for clinical Hemoperfusion

1	ΔA-V sufficient to reverse equilibrium
2	Sorbent has greater drug binding affinity than protein and cells
3	Time dose cytoactivity relationship
4	Drug removal is a significant addition to metabolism, conjugation, and excretion
5	Maximum effective biocompatibility
6	Advantage over established modes of treatment

and produced both consciousness and survival. Dilution is the most primitive method of lowering the plasma concentration of target molecules.

This concept led to the first use of dialysis to reverse barbiturate poisoning [2]. Its subsequent use in a large variety of overdosage and poisoning enabled us to devise standard criteria for the application of dialysis in the removal of drugs [3].

Dialysis, however, is best directed at target molecules with a high unbound fraction in the aqueous phase of plasma (fig. 1). Exemplifying well-accepted pharmacokinetic criteria, the steadily diminishing fraction of drug in plasma as time goes on, makes dialysis less appropriate when there is late referral of patients. In addition, many drugs do not exist in the aqueous phase but are highly lipid soluble or tightly protein bound. We, therefore, devised a resin column more applicable to lipid-soluble or bound drugs [4].

Glutethimide (Doriden) is an excellent example of a drug which is much less dialyzable than phenobarbital and which is highly lipid soluble and concentrates in body fat. A high arteriovenous difference in concentration (ΔA-V) is required to reverse the direction of plasma transport. For this reason we turned early on to the use of charcoal hemoperfusion (fig. 2) for removal of glutethimide [5], digoxin and a host of other bound molecules. In addition to efficacy in providing a high ΔA-V, hemoperfusion has the additional virtue of being quick and potentially widely available to emergency rooms and poison centers.

As we enter a new era of sorbents with designed specificity, a host of new biocompatible coatings and better configurations for our cartridges, it is timely to consider some standard criteria for *hemoperfusion* which are abbreviated in table I.

Several important considerations play a role in the decision making when presented with a patient intoxicated with drugs or chemicals. The target molecule must be present in the blood in a sufficient concentration to provide enough arteriovenous or inlet-outlet difference (Δ A-V) to reverse an equilibrium with cells or tissue. If the target molecule is bound, the sorbent must have greater binding energy or affinity than the critical blood cell or protein. There should be a time-dose cytoactive relationship, i.e. a provable relationship between the blood concentration, the duration of the body's exposure to the chemical and its ultimate biological activity. With poisons and some drugs, this becomes a time-dose cytotoxic relationship. The total amount of target molecule removed must be a significant addition to the natural mechanisms of removal such as metabolism, conjugation and excretion.

Maximum biocompatibility must be sought with minimum impairment of efficiency.

The perfusion procedure must be more rapid, more effective, less dangerous and more available than established modes of removal (e.g. hemodialysis, peritoneal dialysis, hemofiltration, dilution, etc.).

Careful attention to criteria such as these will predictably establish hemoperfusion as a standard life-saving therapeutic procedure and will hasten the day when we will have at our disposal a whole spectrum of sorbent devices, each designed for a specific class of drugs or for a toxic state resulting in coma such as uremia or hepatic failure.

References

1 Cutting, R.A.; Koppanyi, T.: Effect of massive intravenous infusions on the course of barbiturate narcosic. Archs int. Pharmacodyn. Thér. *60:* 395 (1938).

2 Kyle, L.H.; Jegher, H.; Walsh, W.P.; Doolan, P.D.; Wishinsky, H.; Pallotta, A.: The application of hemodialysis to the treatment of barbiturate poisoning. J. clin. Invest. *32:* 364 (1953).

3 Schreiner, G.E.: Dialysis of poisons and drugs. Trans. Am. Soc. artif. internal Organs *16:* 544 (1970).

4 Pallotta, A.: Personal commun.

5 DeMyttenaere, M.H.; Maher, J.F.; Schreiner, G.E.: Hemoperfusion through a charcoal column for glutethimide poisoning. Trans. Am. Soc. artif. internal Organs *13:* 190 (1967).

G.E. Schreiner, MD, Georgetown University Medical Center,
Washington, DC 20007 (USA)

Contr. Nephrol., vol. 29, pp. 11–22 (Karger, Basel 1982)

Hemoperfusion in 1981

Thomas Ming Swi Chang
Artificial Cells and Organs Research Centre,
McGill University, Montreal, P.Q., Canada

Introduction

The problems of charcoal embolism and thrombocytopenia had prevented the routine clinical application of the observation that charcoal can remove endogenous and exogenous toxins from perfusing blood of patients [67]. With the use of the principle of artificial cells [4, 5, 9] to prevent these problems, followed by initial clinical applications in uremia [8], acute intoxication [12] and hepatic coma [10], interests in the clinical use of charcoal hemoperfusion were rekindled. A number of symposia and reviews with emphasis on this topic are available [9, 21, 39, 40, 42, 57, 63]. The present symposium offers another opportunity to assess the present status and future directions of hemoperfusion.

Some Charcoal Hemoperfusion Systems Being Used Clinically in 1981

Using the principle of artificial cells, unlimited extensions in membrane materials and configurations could be used for charcoal hemoperfusion. For instance, we have used nylon, collodion (CAC), heparin benzalkonium complex collodion, albumin-collodion (ACAC), cellulose acetate, radiation grafted heparin-cellulose, silicone and others. The large number of other membrane materials tested in other laboratories have been reviewed elsewhere in detail [9, 21, 39, 40, 42, 57, 63]. In this paper, some of those systems being used clinically at present will be used as examples for discussion.

The albumin-collodion coated activated charcoal (ACAC) or collodion coated activated charcoal (CAC) was developed [6] based on a modification of the earlier collodion technique [4, 9]. This approach has been updated [18] and successfully reproduced by centers in China, Germany, Japan, Russia, USA and other countries. Further developments involved (1) variations in the type of charcoal, and (2) variations in membrane materials. Asahi's Hemasorba system is based on the coating of collodion on petroleum-based spherical charcoal developed by Kureha. Another spherical charcoal from thermosetting resin has also been coated with collodion by Nissho to form the Nipro Hemocarbo system. An extension of membrane material using polyhema coating [3] has been developed industrially as the Hemacol system [63]. This approach has been extended further by using a thinner and more blood compatible modification of acrylic hydrogels [59]. Adsorba 300C is a cellulose coated charcoal system developed by Gambro using a special type of extruded activated charcoal developed in Strathclyde [34, 39]. An ultrathin cellulose coated system developed by Teijin Co. in Japan has also been used clinically [49]. The Detoxifier Type 1 developed recently in Shanghai, China, uses cross-linked gelatin coating with good blood compatibility [66]. In addition, there are many other coated charcoal systems [7, 21, 39, 40, 42, 57, 63]. Other configurations include the Fixed-bed system of Hemodetoxifier of Becton-Dickinson and different types of sorbent membranes of Enka and Gambro [21, 38–40, 42, 57, 63].

Present Status of Different Hemoperfusion Systems

From tables I and II one can make the following comments. (1) Different types of polymer membranes with different permeability characteristics have been used. This results in systems with widely varied permeability characteristics. (2) Membrane thickness varies from 0.05 μm to as thick as 3 μm. When the same membrane material is used, permeability decreases with increasing membrane thickness. With the use of ultrathin membrane (e.g. 0.05 μm), the openings of channels in the charcoal granule are not coated over thus allowing for much better permeability especially to larger molecules. (3) Some systems are very blood compatible whereas others are not. Those which are not blood compatible may deplete platelets or cause platelet aggregates. In addition, cells and fibrin deposits may also decrease the transport rate of those systems which are not blood compatible. In this regard, the actual clearance obtained in the clinical trial is a better index than in vitro clearance using aqueous solution.

The earlier industrial models were developed with emphasis on the safety of the large-scale production. This necessitated the use of thicker membranes and different types of polymers. As experience is gained from these earlier industrial models, ever improving industrially produced systems approaching the ACAC laboratory research model are being produced. As the improved commercial systems replace the less effective commercial systems the clinical results also improve. Unfortunately, in the meantime, a large part of the clinical results accumulated are still based on the use of the earlier commercial models. For example, even though the laboratory system and some of the recent commercial systems

Table I. Some coated charcoal hemoperfusion systems in 1981

System	Membrane Material (thickness)
ACAC and CAC (Chang); Dialaid	albumin-collodion or collodion (0.05 μm)
Hemacol (Smith & Nephew)	acrylic hydrogel (3.00 μm)
Hemodetoxifier (Becton-Dickinson)	fixed-bed charcoal (–)
Adsorba 300C (Gambro)	cellulose (3.00 μm)
Hemasorba (Asahi)	collodion (0.50 μm)
Nipro Hemocarbo (Nissho)	collodion (thin)
Detoxifier Type I (Shanghai)	cross-linked gelatin (?)
HMAC [59]	modified acrylic hydrogel (1.50 μm)
Other coated activated charcoal systems	

Table II. Clinical clearance and blood compatibility of some hemoperfusion systems [17, 21, 23, 39, 44, 49, 50, 57, 59, 64]

	ACAC	Hemacol	Hemodetoxifier	Adsorba 300C	HMAC	Hemasorba
	(Q_B300)	(Q_B300)	(Q_B200)	(Q_B200)	(Q_B250)	(Q_B300)
Middle molecules	144	35	no data	120	31	145
Uric acid	235	94	no data	180	110	230
Creatinine	230	152	100	184	165	230
% of initial platelet	90	70	47	90–96	90–95	90

are blood compatible (table II), the old stigma of platelet depletions using the earlier commercial models persists. The other problem is that as can be seen in table II, some of the older commercial models have much lower clearances for middle molecules, creatinine and uric acid. As the improved commercial systems become available these misconceptions are gradually being resolved.

Hemoperfusion in Chronic Renal Failure

Table III summarizes some of the long-term charcoal hemoperfusion studies in chronic renal failure. In the initial studies carried out here using ACAC hemoperfusion alternating with hemodialysis [8, 9, 11, 14], or with hemoperfusion in series with hemodialysis [16, 19], we have reported improvements in nausea, vomiting, pruritis, feeling of well-being, and improvement in peripheral neuropathy. These results were collaborated by those using a similar system of albu-

Table III. Long-term coated charcoal hemoperfusion in uremia

ACAC-HD	improvements in nausea, vomiting, pruritus, well being [8, 11, 14]
ACAC/HD	improvement in peripheral neuropathy [16]
Hemacol/HD	well tolerated [64]
ACBAC/HD	maintained symptom-free [48]
Hemodetoxifier/HD	no long-term adverse effects [58]
ACAC/UF	improvements in hematocrit, less fluid retention [24, 25]
Adsorba 300C/HD	improvement in pericarditis [45]
CeAC(Teijin)/HD	improvement in pericarditis [49]
ACAC, ACBAC, DHP-1/HD	improvement in peripheral neuropathy [1]
HMAC/HD	improvements in peripheral neuropathy, pruritis, pericarditis, well being [59]

min-collodion coated petroleum-based bead activated charcoal in series with hemodialysis [48]. However, the results reported by groups using Hemacol in series with hemodialysis [44, 64] or Hemodetoxifier in series with hemodialysis [58] were not as enthusiastic.

During this time conflicting laboratory results were also reported. For instance, the high clearance values of the ACAC system for middle molecules, creatinine, uric acid and the protective effect on platelets [8, 9, 11, 13, 14, 16, 17, 48] were not collaborated by others using the older commercial models [44, 58, 64]. It is obvious from table II why some of these discrepancies arise. It also follows that differences in the clearance values obtained in studies of hemoperfusion in series with hemodialysis were obtained too (table IV). With the development of the higher permeability and more biocompatible commercial systems, the results become much clearer. For instance, it was found that the clearance of Adsorba 300C for middle molecules [50], though not as high, is close to that of the ACAC system [8, 14, 19, 23]. Furthermore, platelet removal, as in the case of ACAC, is negligible [50]. Further improvement of commercial system is available in the form of the Hemasorba system using a thin membrane of collodion to coat spherical activated charcoal. It was demonstrated here that the clearance of Hemasorba is comparable to that of theACAC system (table II). With continuing improvements of commercial systems (table I, II, IV), there have been increasing reports of clinical improvements in hematocrit, pericarditis, peripheral neuropathy, pruritis and feeling of well-being [8, 11–14, 19, 23, 24, 45, 48, 59]. In assessing the use of hemoperfusion for chronic renal failure one has to be careful in differentiating the results of those using the older commercial systems and the more recent improved systems.

Two developments that are interesting include (1) the use of hemoperfusion in series with hemodialysis, and (2) the use of hemoperfusion in series with a small ultrafiltrator.

Table IV. Hemoperfusion in series with hemodialysis (HD) or ultrafiltrator (UF) (clearance ml/min)

Solute	ACAC/HD	Hemacol/HD	HMCA/HD	ACAC/UF	Dialad/HFHD	RP-6
	(Q_B300)	(Q_B300)	(Q_B250)	(Q_B300)	(Q_B200)	(Q_B300)
Middle molecules	144	(51)	51	160	160	59
Uric acid	230	165	132	240	–	–
Creatinine	235	275	250	235	230	–
Urea	+++	+++	+++	±	+++	+++
Water + NaCl	++	++	++	+++	+++	+++

Hemoperfusion in Series with Hemodialysis

We have initially demonstrated here that one 2-hour ACAC hemoperfusion-hemodialysis when replaced one of the 6 h, 3 times a week hemodialysis, resulted in improvements in nerve conduction velocity [16]. This approach also solves the problems of electrolyte, urea and fluid removal. This has resulted in much interest in following this combined approach [48–50, 58, 59, 64]. In the most recent large-scale studies carried out in Italy the effectiveness of this approach has been clearly demonstrated [59]. A new development in hemoperfusion-hemodialysis is the 'composite artificial kidney' (CAK) which is the use of a collodion coated activated charcoal hemoperfusion system in series with a high flux capillary hemodialysis membrane [43]. With this combined use, the clearance for middle molecules could be increased to 160 ml/min in clinical trial [43].

Hemoperfusion-Ultrafiltration

Another approach is the combined use of hemoperfusion and a small (0.2 m^2) ultrafiltrator, the latter for the removal of water and sodium chloride [16, 17, 19, 23, 24]. The ultrafiltrator is not used here for hemofiltration because in this approach no hemodialysis equipment is required and the ultrafiltrator is used only to remove and discard all the filtered fluid (up to 2.7 liters) based entirely on the hydrostatic pressure of the blood pump. Long-term clinical trial has demonstrated the safety and effectiveness of this approach [24]. The completion of this system would have to wait for the development of a urea removal system. The use of oral oxystarch in combination with this approach is being tested here. The urea adsorbing capacity of oxystarch [36] could be improved further. Other urea removal systems that have been looked into here include the use of multienzyme systems [25, 68, 69] and the use of conversion of urea to ammonia by urease and the removal of the ammonia as NH_3 gas [51, 52]. The earlier study here of using urease and ammonia adsorbent in microcapsules [5, 9] for oral administration [7, 9, 18] has been developed [32] to a stage where it is now being tested clinically [41].

Table V. Treatment of galactosamine induced fulminant hepatic coma rats

Grade of coma	Type of treatment	Survival time compared to controls	Survival rate compared to controls
II	ACAC hemoperfusion	increased	increased
II	homologous liver perfusion	increased	increased
II	cross circulation	n.s.	n.s.
III	ACAC hemoperfusion	increased	n.s.
III	homologous liver perfusion	n.s.	n.s.
III	fresh blood exchange	n.s.	n.s.
III	ACAC + fresh blood exchange	increased	n.s.
III	ACAC + glucagon + insulin	n.s.	n.s.
III	2 × ACAC + fresh blood exchange	increased	increased

Hemoperfusion in Liver failure

The observation that hemoperfusion can result in the temporary recovery of consciousness in grade IV hepatic coma patients [10, 13, 17, 19] is now conclusive [1, 2, 21, 33, 35, 40, 57, 63]. However, its effect on long-term survival has not yet been established. A galactosamine-induced fulminant hepatic coma rat model has been used here to study in detail the effects of charcoal hemoperfusion on the survival rates of the animals [22, 31, 46, 60]. The results are summarized in table V. In grade II coma rats, ACAC hemoperfusion has been conclusively demonstrated to increase both the survival time and the survival rate [22, 31, 60]. Detailed studies carried out using ACAC in galactosamine-induced FHF rats by another laboratory also show very similar results [47]. We have found that homologous liver perfusion but not cross-circulation resulted in significant increases in survival time and survival rate of grade II coma rats [46]. ACAC hemoperfusions carried out in grade III coma rats only increased the survival time but not the survival rate [22, 60]. Homologous liver perfusions are not effective in increasing either the survival time or the survival rate of grade III coma rats [46]. This raises the question that perhaps it is not the artificial liver support system that is not adequate. Further study was carried out to see whether the use of fresh blood exchange transfusion and possible hepatotropic agents may increase the survival rates [22, 60]. The results obtained showed that in Grade III coma, hemoperfusion only increased the survival time but not the survival rate, unless a regime of multiple hemoperfusions plus fresh blood exchange was used [22, 60].

One cannot transfer the results in rats directly to patients. For instance the survival rate in control untreated grade II coma rats is about 30% and that of grade III coma rats in 0–2%. Thus, the survival rates of grade II coma rats is more comparable to grade III coma in patients. Since the publication of our studies showing the effectiveness of ACAC hemoperfusion in FHF rats in earlier grades of coma [22, 31], one group in the United Kingdom has been starting to treat patients in grade III coma with charcoal hemoperfusion [35].

Charcoal Hemoperfusion in Acute Intoxication

ACAC hemoperfusion has resulted in high clearance and recovery of patients with acute intoxication [12, 19, 26]. Patients with the following drug intoxication have been treated successfully here using ACAC with clearance as shown (table VI): glutethimide 230 (Q_B300); phenobarbital 228 (Q_B300); methyprylon 230 (Q_B300); methaqualone 230 (Q_B300); salicylate 150 (Q_B300); secobarbital 200 (Q_B230) and theophylline 90 (Q_B90). The use of charcoal hemoperfusion in acute intoxication has been the subject of many discussions. Some of these have been summarized [17, 19, 21, 26, 36, 39, 42, 57]. It would appear that most people agree that charcoal hemoperfusion has a role in the treatment of severely poisoned patients if the drug in question does not have a large volume distribution. The question of whether charcoal hemoperfusion is useful in drugs with large volume distribution is still under study [57]. Hemoperfusion has also been used successfully for the treatment of acute intoxication in small pediatric patients [27, 30].

Albumin in Hemoperfusion

Albumin was applied to the CAC system to form the more blood compatible system of ACAC [6, 8, 9, 15, 18]. It was found that this albumin coating on the membrane also functions as a carrier and binder for some molecules [21]. Table VI summarizes some of the other applications. The subsequent uses of albumin for making other hemoperfusion systems more blood compatible include its use on resins [57, 62], and on synthetic immunosorbents [28]. This albumin-coating approach may greatly increase the clinical applications of these and other adsorbents and immunosorbents by making them more blood compatible. Albumin-collodion activated charcoal removes a small amount of bilirubin [9, 10]. Other investigators found that by entrapping more albumin in particles, much more bilirubin can be removed in hemoperfusion. Using the ACAC system from here [6], it was found that albumin in this system can be used to remove anti-albumin from perfusing plasma [61], this has led to the use of antigens or antibodies entrapped in the collodion charcoal system for immunosorbent [36, 61].

Table VI. Drug clearance using ACAC

Drugs	Initial clearance, ml/min	Blood flow, ml/min
Glutethimide	230	300
Phenobarbital	228	300
Methyprylon	230	300
Methaqualone	230	300
Salicylate	150	300
Secobarbital	200	230
Theophylline	90	90 (pediatric)

Hemoperfusion Using Resins, Immobilized Enzymes, Immunosorbents and Other Systems

Charcoal hemoperfusion, being widely used clinically, is discussed in detail here for acute intoxication, uremia and liver failure. There are many other possible applications [21, 57, 65].

Hemoperfusion with anionic exchange resin has been rested in vitro for diabetic ketoacidosis [37]. Other adsorbents [54], enzymes and other biologically active materials for hemoperfusion are described elsewhere [9, 20, 53, 57]. For example, an albumin-collodion coated synthetic immunosorbent system can efficiently remove blood group anti-A and anti-B [28]. An albumin coated immunosorbent of this type has already been tested recently in another center in clinical trials for the removal of blood group antibodies for bone marrow transplantation. With the initial demonstration that microencapsulated enzyme can be used in hemoperfusion to act on substrate in the blood [5], many other immobilized enzyme systems have been used for hemoperfusion [9, 20, 29]. More recently, artificial cells containing tyrosine have been used here successfully in hemoperfusions to lower tyrosine and phenols in hepatic coma rats [55, 56]. With the development of artificial cells containing multienzyme systems [20, 25], especially the recent development of lipid-polymer membrane systems to retain substrates and cofactors [68, 69], more complex metabolic hemoperfusion systems will be available on the horizon.

Summary

The present status of hemoperfusion using the principle of artificial cells is described in detail using coated charcoal hemoperfusion as an example. The laboratory and clinical results show that in 1981 increasing numbers of new commercial models are approaching the efficiency and blood compatibility of the ACAC laboratory system. The results of hemoperfusion for uremia, acute intoxication and hepatic coma are analyzed. Other approaches are briefly discussed.

References

1 Agishi, T.; Yamashita, N.; Ota, K.: Clinical results of direct charcoal hemoperfusion for endogenous and exogenous intoxication; in Sideman, Chang, Hemoperfusion: Kidney and liver support and detoxification, part I, pp. 255–263 (Hemisphere, Washington 1980).

2 Amano, I.; Kano, H.; Takahira, H.; Yamamoto, Y.; Itoh, K.; Iwatsuki, S.; Maeda, K.; Ohta, K.: Hepatic assist system using bead-type charcoal; in Chang, Artificial kidney, artificial liver, and artificial cells, pp. 89–98 (Plenum Press, New York 1978).

3 Andrade, J.D.; Wagenen, R. van; Ghavamian, M.; Voder, J.; Kirkham, R.; Kolff, W.J.: Coated adsorbent for direct blood perfusion. Trans. Am. Soc. artif. internal Organs *18:* 235 (1972).

4 Chang, T.M.S.: Semipermeable microcapsules. Science *146:* 524–525 (1964).

5 Chang, T.M.S.: Semipermeable aqueous microcapsules ('artificial cells'): with emphasis on experiments in an extracorporeal shunt system. Trans. Am. Soc. artif. internal Organs *12:* 13–19 (1966).

6 Chang, T.M.S.: Removal of endogenous and exogenous toxins by a microencapsulated absorbent. Can. J. Physiol. Pharmacol. *47:* 1043–1045 (1969).

7 Chang, T.M.S.; Loa, S.K.: Urea removal by urease and ammonia adsorbent in the intestine. Physiologist *13:* 70 (1970).

8 Chang, T.M.S.; Gonda, A.; Dirks, J.H.; Malave, N.: Clinical evaluation of chronic, intermittent, and short term hemoperfusions in patients with chronic renal failure using semipermeable microcapsules (artificial cells) formed from membrane-coated activated charcoal. Trans. Am. Soc. artif. internal Organs *17:* 246–252 (1971).

9 Chang, T.M.S.: Artificial cells (Thomas, Springfield 1972).

10 Chang, T.M.S.: Haemoperfusions over microencapsulated adsorbent in a patient with hepatic coma. Lancet *ii:* 1371–1372 (1972).

11 Chang, T.M.S.; Gonda, A.; Dirks, J.H.; Coffey, J.F.; Burns, T.: ACAC microcapsule artificial kidney for the long term and short term management of eleven patients with chronic renal failure. Trans. Am. Soc. artif. internal Organs *18:* 465–472 (1972).

12 Chang, T.M.S.; Coffey, J.F.; Lister, C.; Taroy, E.; Stark, A.: Methaqualone, methyprylon, and glutethimide clearance by the ACAC microcapsule artificial kidney: in vitro and in patients with acute intoxication. Trans. Am. Soc. artif. internal Organs *19:* 87–91 (1973).

13 Chang, T.M.S.; Migchelsen, M.: Characterization of possible 'toxic' metabolites in uremia and hepatic coma based on the clearance spectrum for larger molecules by ACAC microcapsule artificial kidney. Trans. Am. Soc. artif. internal Organs *19:* 314–319 (1973).

14 Chang, T.M.S.; Migchelsen, M., Coffey, J.F.; Stark, A.: Serum middle molecule levels in uremia during long term intermittent hemoperfusions with the ACAC (coated charcoal) microcapsule artificial kidney. Trans. Am. Soc. artif. internal Organs *20:* 364–371 (1974).

15 Chang, T.M.S.: Platelet-surface interaction: effect of albumin coating or heparin complexing on thrombogenic surfaces. Can. J. Physiol. Pharmacol. *52:* 275–285 (1974).

16 Chang, T.M.S.; Chirito, E.; Barre, P.; Cole, C.; Hewish, M.: Clinical performance characteristics of a new combined system for simultaneous hemoperfusion-hemodialysis-ultrafiltration in series. Trans. Am. Soc. artif. internal Organs *21:* 502–508 (1975).

17 Chang, T.M.S.: Microencapsulated adsorbent hemoperfusion for uremia, intoxication and hepatic failure. Kidney int. *7:* S387–S392 (1975).

18 Chang, T.M.S.: Microcapsule artificial kidney: including updated preparative procedures and properties. Kidney int. *10:* S218–S224 (1976).
19 Chang, T.M.S.: Hemoperfusion alone and in series with ultrafiltration or dialysis for uremia, poisoning and liver failure. Kidney int. *10:* S305–S311 (1976).
20 Chang, T.M.S.: Biomedical applications of immobilized enzymes and proteins, vol. 1, 2 (Plenum Press, New York 1977).
21 Chang, T.M.S.: Artificial kidney, artificial liver, and artificial cells (Plenum Press, New York 1978).
22 Chang, T.M.S.; Lister, C.; Chirito, E.; O'Keefe, P.; Resurreccion, E.: Effects of hemoperfusion rate and time of initiation of ACAC charcoal hemoperfusion on the survival of fulminant hepatic failure rats. Trans. Am. Soc. artif. internal Organs *24:* 243–245 (1978).
23 Chang, T.M.S.: Assessments of clinical trials of charcoal hemoperfusion in uremic patients. Clin. Nephrol. *11:* 111–119 (1979).
24 Chang, T.M.S.; Chirito, E.; Barre, P.; Cole, C.; Lister, C.; Resurreccion, E.: Long-term clinical assessment of combined ACAC hemoperfusion-ultrafiltration in uremia. Artif. Organs *3:* 127–131 (1979).
25 Chang, T.M.S.; Malouf, C.; Resurreccion, E.: Artificial cells containing multienzyme systems for the sequential conversion of urea into ammonia, glutamate, then alanine. Artif. Organs *3:* S284–S287 (1979).
26 Chang, T.M.S.: Clinical experience with ACAC coated charcoal hemoperfusion in acute intoxication. Clin. Toxicol. *17:* 529–542 (1980).
27 Chang, T.M.S.; Espinosa-Melendez, E.; Francoeur, T.E.; Eade, N.R.: Albumin-collodion activated coated charcoal hemoperfusion in the treatment of severe theophylline intoxication in a 3-year-old patient. Pediatrics, Springfield *65:* 811–814 (1980).
28 Chang, T.M.S.: Blood compatible coating of synthetic immunoadsorbents. Trans. Am. Soc. artif. internal Organs *26:* 546–549 (1980).
29 Chang, T.M.S.: Artificial cells: the use of hybrid systems. Artif. Organs *4:* 264–271 (1980).
30 Chavers, B.M.; Kjellstrand, C.M.; Wiegand, C.; Ebben, J.; Mauer, S.M.: Techniques for use of charcoal hemoperfusion in infants: experience in two patients. Kidney Int. *18:* 386 (1980).
31 Chirito, E.; Reiter, B.; Lister, C.; Chang, T.M.S.: Artificial liver: The effect of ACAC microencapsulated charcoal hemoperfusion on fulminant hepatic failure. Artif. Organs *1:* 76–83 (1977).
32 Gardner, D.L.; Falb, R.D.; Kim, B.C.; Emmerling, D.C.: Possible uremic detoxification via oral ingested microcapsules. Trans. Am. Soc. artif. internal Organs *17:* 239 (1971).
33 Gelfand, M.C.; Winchester, J.F.; Knepshield, J.H.; Cohan, S.L.; Schreiner, G.E.: Biochemical correlates of reversal of hapatic coma coated with charcoal hemoperfusion. Trans. Am. Soc. artif. internal Organs *24:* 239–342 (1978).
34 Gilchrist, T.: Reflections on the role of carbon hemaadsorption in therapeutic medicine. Contr. Nephrol., vol. 29, pp. 34–52 (Karger, Basel 1982).
35 Gimson, A.E.S.; Hughes, R.D.; Langley, P.G.: Canalese, J.; Williams, R.: King's experience with artificial liver support; in Sideman, Chang, Hemoperfusion: Kidney and liver support and detoxification, part I, pp. 285–294 (Hemisphere, Washington 1980).
36 Giordano, C.: Sorbents and their clinical applications (Academic Press, New York 1979).
37 Giordano, C.; Esposito, R.; Bello, P.; Quarto, E.; Cirillo, D.; Pluvio, M.; Lauzetti, N.; Calabria, L.: Hemoperfusion in diabetic coma. Contr. Nephrol., vol. 29, pp. 82–89 (Karger, Basel 1982).

38 Gurland, H.J.; Castro, L.A.; Hillebrand, G.; Schmidt, B.: Sorbent membranes and their medical applications; in Sideman, Chang, Hemoperfusion: Kidney and liver support and detoxification, part 1, pp. 105–110 (Hemisphere, Washington 1980).
39 Kennedi, R.M.; Courtney, J.M.; Gaylor, J.D.S.; Gilchrist, T.: Artificial organs (MacMillan, London 1977).
40 Kikolaef, V.G.; Strelko, V.V.: Hemoperfusion (Naukova Dumka, Kiev 1979).
41 Kjellstrand, C.; Borges, H.; Pru, C.; Gardner, D.; Fink, D.: Urease-zirconium-phosphate microcapsules (UZP) effectively decreases nitrogen accumulation in CRF patients (Abstract). Am. Soc. artif. internal Organs *10:* 47 (1981).
42 Klinkmann, H.; Falkenhagen, D.; Courtney, J.M.: Blood purification by hemoperfusion. Int. J. artif. Organs *2:* 296 (1979).
43 Lacaille, Y.; Chang, T.M.S.; Picart, X.; Lobel, A.; Messier, D.; Man, N.K.: CAK – composite artificial kidney. Abstr., III Congr. Int. Soc. Artif. Organs, Paris 1980.
44 Leber, H.W.; Neuhauser, M.; Goubeaud, G.: Hemoperfusion versus hemodialysis in uremia: biochemical analysis. Eur. Soc. artif. Organs *3:* 202 (1976).
45 Martin, A.M.; Gibbins, T.K.; Kimmit, T.; Rennie, F.: Hemodialysis and hemoperfusion in the treatment of uremic pericarditis. A study of 13 cases. Dial. Transplant. *8:* 135 (1979).
46 Mohsini, K.; Lister, C.; Chang, T.M.S.: The effects of homologous cross circulation and in situ liver perfusion on fulminant hepatic failure rats. Artif. Organs *4:* 171–175 (1980).
47 Niu, Z.; Jia, S.R.; Zhang, D.Y.; Xu, C.X.; Tang, X.J.; Fan, W.K.; Luo, Y.P.; Li, Z.M.: The effects of hemoperfusion in galactosamine induced FHF rats. Chungking med. College Bull. *November:* 1–6 (1980).
48 Odaka, M.; Tabata, Y.; Kobayashi, H.; Nomura, Y.; Soma, H.; Hirasawa, H.; Sato, H.: Clinical experience of bead-shaped charcoal haemoperfusion in chronic renal failure and fulminant hepatic failure; in Chang, Artificial kidney, artificial liver, and artificial cells, pp. 79–88 (Plenum Press, New York 1978).
49 Odaka, M.; Hirasawa, H.; Kobayashi, H.; Ohkawa, M.; Soeda, K.; Tabata, Y.; Soma, M.; Sato, H.: Clinical and fundamental studies of cellulose coated bead-shaped charcoal haemoperfusion in chronic renal failure; in Sideman, Chang, Hemoperfusion: kidney and liver support and detoxification, part I, pp. 45–55 (Hemisphere, Washington 1980).
50 Oules, R.; Asaba, H.; Neuhauser, M.; Yahiel, V.; Baehrendtz, S.; Gunnarsson, B.; Bergstrom, J.; Furst, P.: Hemoperfusion and removal of endogenous uremic middle molecules; in Chang, Artificial kidney, artificial liver, and artificial cells, pp. 153–164 (Plenum Press, New York 1978).
51 Pişkin, E.; Chang, T.M.S.: Urea and ammonium removal based on alkalinization and removal of free ammonia. Int. J. artif. Organs *2:* 211–214 (1979).
52 Pişkin, E.; Chang, T.M.S.: Effects of temperature on the removal of urea as ammonia by enzyme conversion and gas absorption using an oxygenator. Int. J. artif. Organs *4:* 45–48 (1981).
53 Pişkin, K.; Chang, T.M.S.: A new combined enzyme-charcoal system formed by enzyme adsorption on charcoal followed by polymer coating. Int. J. artif. Organs *3:* 344–347 (1980).
54 Rosenbaum, J.L.: Experience with resin hemoperfusion; in Chang, Artificial kidney, artificial liver, and artificial cells, pp. 217–214 (Plenum Press, New York 1978).
55 Shu, C.D.; Chang, T.M.S.: Tyrosinase immobilized within artificial cells for detoxification in liver failure. I. Preparation and in vitro studies. Int. J. Artif. Organs *3:* 287–291 (1980).

56 Shu, C.D.; Chang, T.M.S.: Tyrosinase immobilized within artificial cells for detoxification in liver failure. II. In vivo studies in fulminant hepatic failure rats. Int. J. artif. Organs *4:* 82–84 (1981).
57 Sideman, S.; Chang, T.M.S.: Hemoperfusion: Kidney and liver support and detoxification, part I (Hemisphere, Washington 1980).
58 Siemsen, A.W.; Dunea, G.; Maindani, B.H.; Guruprakash, G.: Charcoal hemoperfusion in chronic renal failure. Nephron *22:* 386 (1978).
59 Stefoni, S.; Coli, L.; Feliciangeli, G.; Baldrati, L.; Bonomini, V.: Regular hemoperfusion in regular dialysis treatment. A long-term study. Int. J. artif. Organs *3:* 348 (1980).
60 Tabata, Y.; Chang, T.M.S.: Comparisons of six artificial liver support regimes in fulminant hepatic coma rats. Trans. Am. Soc. artif. internal Organs *26:* 394–399 (1980).
61 Terman, D.S.; Tavel, T.; Petty, D.; Racic, M.R.; Buffaloe, G.: Specific removal of antibody by extracorporeal circulation over antigen immobilized in collodion charcoal. Clin. exp. Immunol. *28:* 180 (1977).
62 Ton, H,-Y.; Hughes, R.D.; Silk, D.B.A.; Williams, R.: Albumin-coated amberlite XAD-7 resin for hemoperfusion in acute liver failure. Artif. Organs *3:* 20 (1979).
63 Williams, R.; Murray-Lyon, I.M.: Artificial liver support (Pitman, London 1975).
64 Winchester, J.F.; Apiliga, M.T,. MacKay, J.M.; Kennedy, A.C.: Short term evaluation of charcoal hemoperfusion combined with dialysis in uremic patients. Kidney Int. *10:* S315 (1976).
65 Winchester, J.F.; Rahman, A.; Bregman, H.; Mortensen, L.M.; Gelfand, M.C.; Schein, P.S.; Schreiner, G.E.: Role of hemoperfusion in anticancer drug removal; in Sideman, Chang, Hemoperfusion. Kidney and liver support and detoxification, part I, pp. 369–377 (Hemisphere, Washington 1980).
66 Wu, Z.G.; Cai, Z.H.; Wu, G.H.; Qin, X.Y.; Shi, Z.Q.: Clinical applications of artificial liver, artificial kidney and detoxifier type I. Acta acad. Med. Primae, Shanghai *7:* 321–327 (1980).
67 Yatzidis, D.: A convenient hemoperfusion microapparatus and charcoal for the treatment of endogenous and exogenous intoxication. Proc. Eur. Dial. Transplant. Ass. *1:* 83 (1964).
68 Yu, Y.T.; Chang, T.M.S.: Ultrathin lipid-polymer membrane microcapsules containing multienzymes, cofactors and substrates for multistep enzyme reactions. FEBS Lett. *125:* 94–96 (1981).
69 Yu, Y.T.; Chang, T.M.S.: Lipid-polymer membrane artificial cells containing multienzyme systems, cofactors and substrates for the removal of ammonia and urea. Trans. Am. Soc. artif. internal Organs (1981).

Prof. T.M.S. Chang, Artificial Cells and Organs Research Centre, McGill University, H3G 1Y6 Montreal, Que. (Canada)

Contr. Nephrol., vol. 29, pp. 23–33 (Karger, Basel 1982)

In Vitro Assessment of Charcoal and Resin Hemoadsorbents

D. Falkenhagen, S. Gottschall, G. Esther, J.M. Courtney, H. Klinkmann

Department of Medicine, Wilhelm Pieck University, Rostock, GDR, and
Bioengineering Unit, University of Strathclyde, Glasgow, UK

Introduction

The possible advantages arising from the successful use of adsorbents in blood purification have stimulated activity in the clinical assessment of hemoperfusion in the areas of acute poisoning, liver failure and uremia [10]. However, this assessment has not eliminated the need for adequate preclinical evaluation of potential hemoadsorbents, since the future role of hemoperfusion has still to be determined. In acute poisoning, there is uncertainty regarding the effectiveness of hemoperfusion for the removal of substances which are mainly tissue bound and results obtained in the treatment of liver failure and uremia [3, 7, 14] do not provide definite conclusions on the usefulness of hemoadsorbents in these areas.

At this stage, it seems reasonable to predict that interest will continue not only in adsorbents of the type already used clinically, but also in approaches involving the combination of adsorbents with other blood purification techniques [8, 13] and the use of more selective adsorbents [1, 11].

The development of hemoadsorbents requires the establishment of suitable in vitro and in vivo test procedures for the assessment of blood compatibility and efficiency. In addition, joint consideration of blood compatibility and efficiency is necessary for the optimization of the properties of the hemoadsorbents. These points have influenced the design of the in vitro evaluation procedures which are described here.

Material and Methods

Charcoals

Designations used for the charcoals in the figures and tables are given in parentheses following the description of that material.

Norit RBX1, a peat-based, extruded charcoal [4] was supplied by Norit-Clydesdale Ltd, UK. The granules were used uncoated (Norit RBX1) or coated with 2.5 cellulose acetate [5] to give a coating weight of 0.5% (Norit RBX1 0.5%) or 1.0% (Norit RBX1 1.0%).

Petroleum-based, spherical charcoal produced by Mitsubishi was taken from the Detoxyl 2 column of Sorin Biomedica, Italy. The granules were uncoated (Mitsubishi).

Petroleum-based, spherical charcoal, used in the Hemosorba device of Asahi, Japan, was supplied by Kimal Scientific Products Ltd, UK. The granules were used uncoated (Asahi uncoated) or coated with collodion to an estimated thickness of 0.5 μm (Asahi coated).

Coconut-based charcoal was taken from the Haemocol device of Smith and Nephew Ltd, UK. The granules were coated with 2–4% of an acrylic hydrogel (Haemocol).

Coconut-based charcoal, used in the Haemocol 100 device and of smaller particle size than the granules used in the Haemocol, was supplied by Smith and Nephew Ltd. The granules were used uncoated (Haemocol fine uncoated) or coated with 2–4% of acrylic hydrogel (Haemocol fine coated).

Resins

XAD-4, a macroreticular resin derived from poly (styrene-divinylbenzene) was taken from the Haemoresin column of Braun, FRG. The adsorbent has a pore size of 5 nm and an active surface area of 750 m^2/g dry weight.

Y56, a macroreticular resin based on poly(styrene-divinylbenzene), was produced by Chemiekombinat, Bitterfeld, GDR, with a pore size of 8 nm and an active surface area of 500 m^2/g. The Y56 resin was coated with human serum albumin (HSA) supplied by VEB Serumwerk Dessau, GDR. HSA concentrations of 0.03, 0.1, 1.0, 5.0 and 10.0 g/100 ml were used. The adsorption rate of HSA calculated for the outer surface of 140.05 cm^2/g dry weight [6] is shown in figure 1 for HSA concentrations of 0.1, 1.0, 2.0 and 5.0 g/100 ml. HSA adsorption was measured using 70 ml of a buffered solution and adjusting to a specific radioactivity of 1.3 MBq/L (fig. 2).

Carbonized resin was obtained by pyrolysis and carbonization of macroreticular resin based on poly(styrene-divinylbenzene).

Agarose Beads

To provide a material for comparison, agarose beads were produced by a modified version of the procedure reported by *Holloway* et al. [9].

Platelet and Leucocyte Assessment

A closed test circuit (fig. 3) was used. The circuit comprised a polypropylene column with a polyurethane filter and a roller pump (Infusomat, Braun, FRG). The column contained 2 g or 2 ml of adsorbent and the circuit operated on a blood volume of 20 ml. Fresh heparinized blood (3 U/ml) was donated by normal male or female volunteers who had not taken antiplatelet drugs for at least 4 weeks prior to the experiment. Before priming the circuit with blood, a heparin solution (5,000 U/l) was introduced. Platelet and leucocyte counts were determined immediately before and after the perfusion time of 120 min. Results were expressed as the percentage fall in platelet or leucocyte levels.

Adsorption of Fibrinogen

This was measured using a buffered solution containing 0.2 g/l fibrinogen (Kabi, Sweden). ^{125}I-fibrinogen (The Radiochemical Centre, Amersham, UK) was added to give a specific activity of 1.3 MBq/L. 70 ml of this solution were introduced to a closed test circuit (fig. 2) and the specific activity of the charged column was determined after 4 h with a gamma counter [6].

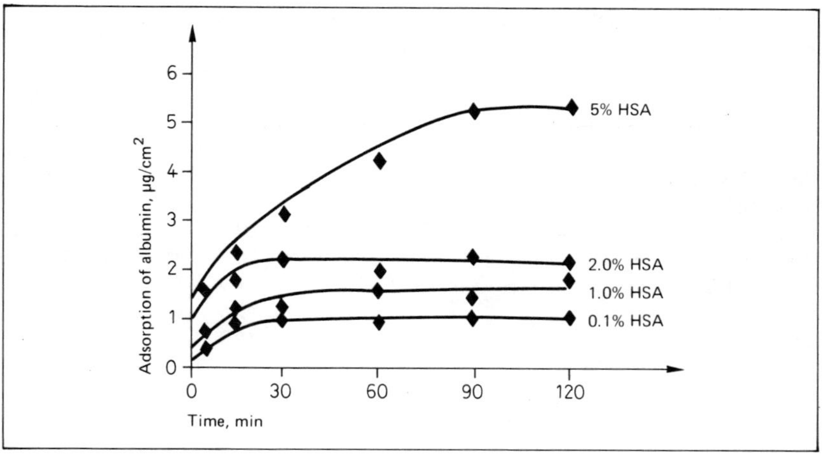

Fig. 1. Adsorption of albumin for the Y56 resin using different concentrations of albumin (n = 3).

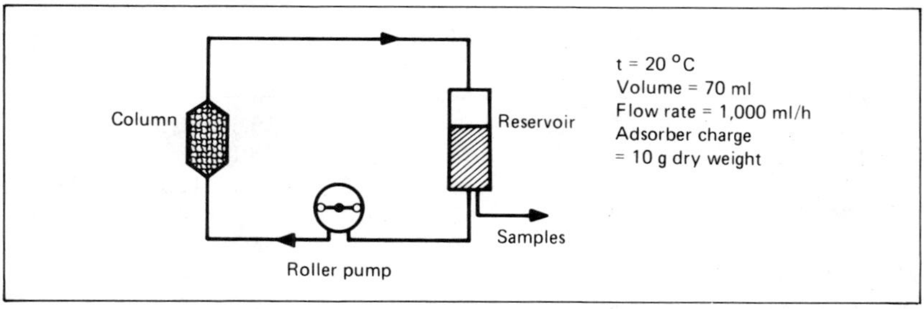

Fig. 2. Test circuit for measuring the adsorption rate of albumin and fibrinogen.

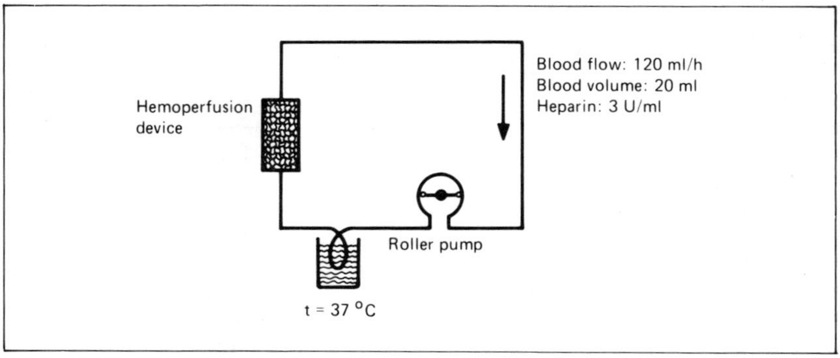

Fig. 3. Diagram of test circuit.

Table I. Fall of platelets and leucocytes using different hemoadsorbents in vitro (2 g dry weight)

Active charcoal	Leucocytes	Platelets
Mitsubishi	10.6 ± 12.7	17.9 ± 9.2
Norit RBX1 uncoated	49.4 ± 8.1	74.4 ± 8.0
Norit RBX1 1.0%	61.3 ± 21.5	26.6 ± 8.2
Haemocol	41.5 ± 10.7	34.2 ± 22.1
Haemocol fine uncoated	52.8 ± 16.4	85.7 ± 3.7
Haemocol fine coated	51.8 ± 7.9	53.5 ± 15.9
XAD-4[1]	66.1 ± 9.8	56.6 ± 24.6
Agarose (4%)[1]	32.2 ± 25.9	22.3 ± 9.8

[1] Wet weight.

Table II. Influence of albumin coating on the in vitro fall in the level of platelets and leucocytes caused by hemoperfusion over uncoated and coated Y56

Absorbent	Platelets		Leucocytes	
	fall %	adsorption $2 \times 10^4/cm^2$	fall %	adsorption $2 \times 10^4/cm^2$
Y56 uncoated	57.7 ± 16.3	664 ± 187	59.3 ± 11.0	34.1 ± 6.2
Y56 0.03% HSA	47.7 ± 10.4	541 ± 195	50.1 ± 13.6	29.0 ± 7.8
Y56 0.1% HSA	48.7 ± 16.4	560 ± 188	56.9 ± 12.2	32.4 ± 7.0
Y56 1.0% HSA	30.6 ± 19.1	351 ± 219	59.1 ± 8.1	34.0 ± 4.6
Y56 5.0% HSA	26.9 ± 9.7	309 ± 112	56.7 ± 11.3	31.8 ± 6.5
Y56 10.0 % HSA	28.6 ± 12.3	329 ± 141	57.2 ± 10.1	32.4 ± 5.8
Empty column (n = 13)	1.8 ± 8.1	–	1.5 ± 11	–

Hemoperfusion time 120 min. n = 6.

Table III. Fibrinogen adsorption of different hemoadsorbents (n = 3)

Adsorbent	Adsorption rate, µg/cm²
Mitsubishi uncoated	12.6
Asahi uncoated	16.9
Asahi coated	7.0
Norit RBX1 uncoated	19.6
Norit RBX1 1% coated	13.9
Y56 uncoated	3.51
Y56 1% HSA	0.74
Y56 5% HSA	1.03
XAD 4 uncoated	2.69

Table IV. Influence of different coatings on the vitamin B_{12} clearance calculated for 100 g of the absorbent (dry weight ml/min)

Albumin coating		Ultrathin polymer coating		Polymer coating	
Y56 uncoated	80.0	Asahi uncoated	111.8	Norit RBX1 uncoated	65
Y56 2% HSA	64.5	Asahi coated	75.2	Norit RBX1 0.25%	24
Y56 5% HSA	42.0			Norit RBX1 0.5%	25
				Norit RBX1 1%	9
				Haemocol	6.4

Flow rate = 1 liter/h. n = 3.

Vitamin B_{12} Clearance

The test circuit was the same as that used for albumin and fibrinogen adsorption (fig. 2). The concentration of vitamin B_{12} (VEB Jenapharm, GDR) was adjusted to 0.1 g/l. ^{58}Co-vitamin B_{12} (Isocommerz, GDR) was added to give a specific activity of 740 KBq/l. 1-ml samples were withdrawn after 5, 15, 30, 60, 90 and 120 min for measurement of specific activity. The vitamin B_{12} clearance of the column was estimated for 100 g of the adsorbent within the first 5 min.

Measurement of Drug Adsorption

200 ml saline containing 150 mg/l of the drug being investigated and 1 g dry weight of the adsorbent were shaken together. Samples were withdrawn after 2 and 6 h and the concentration of the drug measured using of Specord UV VIS (VEB Zeiss Jena, GDR).

Results

Blood Compatibility

Table I lists the alteration in platelet and leucocyte levels induced by different adsorbents. Table II gives the results obtained with Y56 resin, uncoated and coated with albumin and those obtained with an empty column control. Adsorption of platelets and leucocytes, calculated from the fall in platelet and leucocyte levels, is also given. In the calculation, the adsorbent surface was estimated using geometrical parameters [6]. The adsorption rate of fibrinogen for uncoated and coated adsorbents is shown in table III, with the adsorption rate estimated in terms of the outer surface only.

Adsorbent Efficiency

The influence on vitamin B_{12} clearance of coating adsorbents with albumin or polymer is seen in table IV. Figure 4 shows the relationship between vitamin B_{12} removal and charcoal adsorbents. Figure 5 shows the relationship for Y56 resin, uncoated and coated with albumin. The efficiency of adsorbents for the removal of drugs important in acute poisioning is demonstrated in figures 6 and 7.

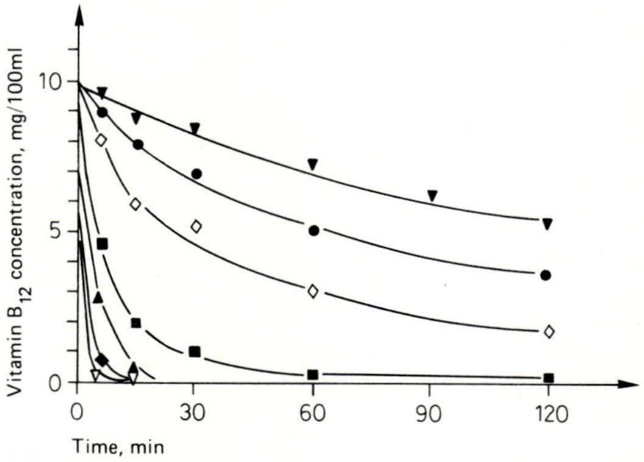

Fig. 4. Decrease of the vitamin B_{12} concentration using different active charcoals in vitro. 70 ml vitamin B_{12} solution, 10 g active charcoal, flow rate = 1 liter/h. ▼ = Haemocol; ■ = Norit RBX1; ◇ = Norit RBX 0.5%; ● = Norit RBX 1.0%; ▲ = Asahi coated; ◆ = Mitsubishi; ▽ = Asahi uncoated.

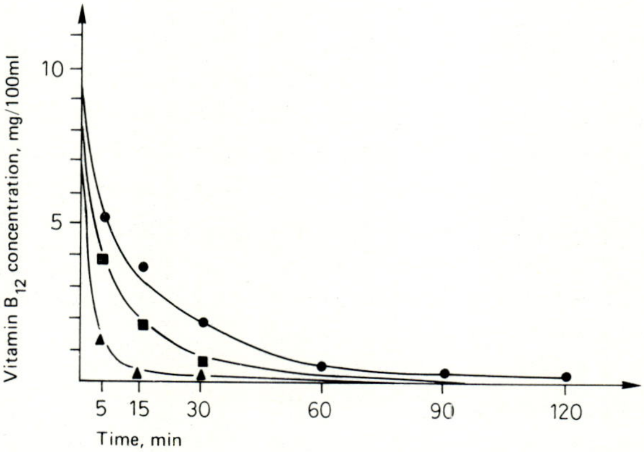

Fig. 5. Decrease of the vitamin B_{12} concentration for Y56 resin uncoated and coated with albumin (HSA). 70 ml vitamin B_{12} solution, 10 g dry weight of Y56, flow rate 1 liter/h. ● = 5% HSA; ■ = 2% HSA; ▲ = uncoated.

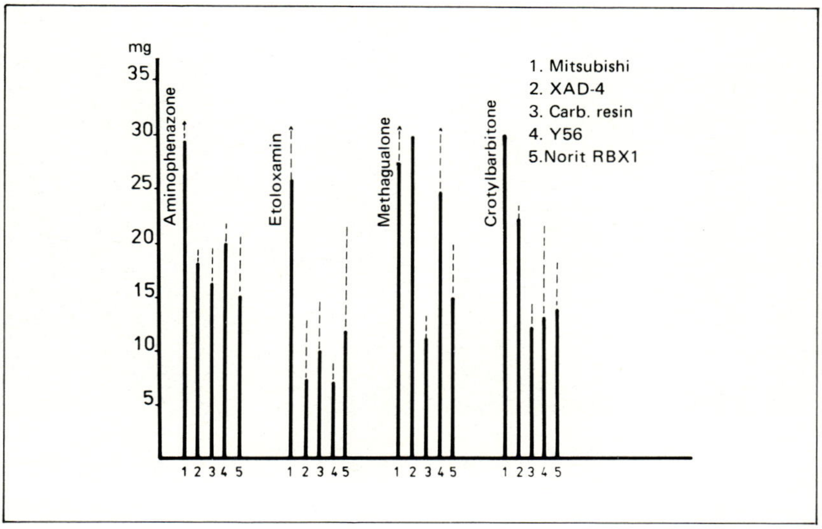

Fig. 6. Adsorption efficiency of different materials for drugs with reference to 1 g dry weight after 2 and 6 h (– – –).

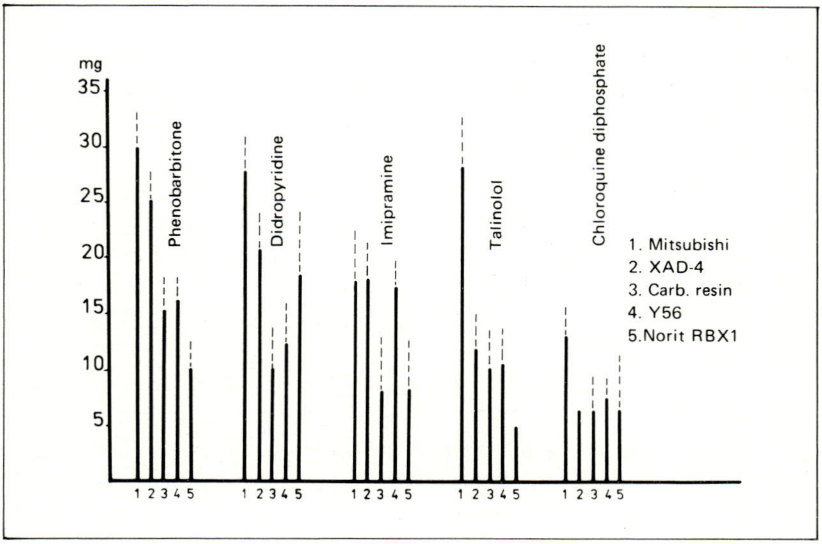

Fig. 7. Adsorption efficiency of different materials for drugs with reference to 1 g dry weight after 2 and 6 h (– – –).

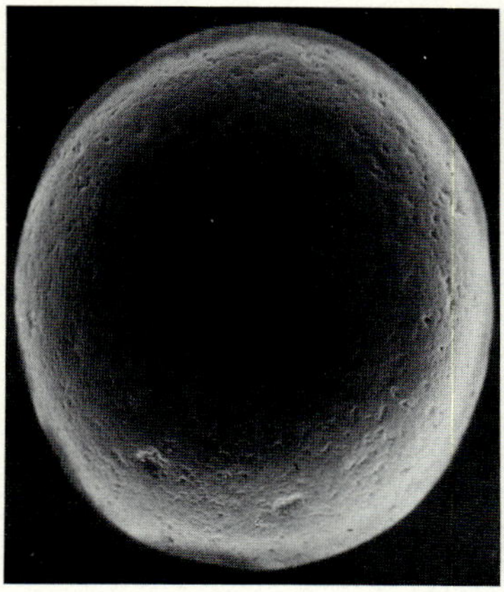
8

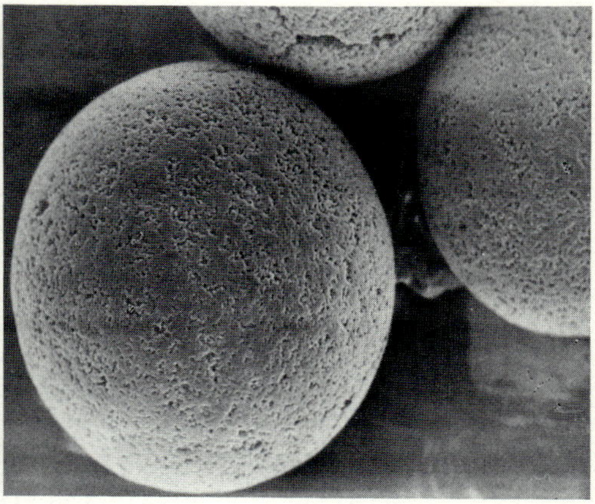
9

Fig. 8. Uncoated Mitsubishi petroleum-based active charcoal. Scanning electron micrograph.

Fig. 9. Uncoated Asahi petroleum-based active charcoal. Scanning electron micrograph.

Discussion

The test circuit designed to study platelet and leucocyte behavior requires only 20 ml of human blood. An important feature is that while a control investigation with an empty column (table II) gave only a negligible decrease in platelets and leucocyte levels, the test circuit detected marked differences in the influence of adsorbents on these levels.

The Mitsubishi spherical charcoal used in the Sorin Detoxyl 2 column was the most promising adsorbent in terms of its effect on platelets and leucocytes. This is an agreement with results obtained during an investigation of hemoperfusion in the rat [12]. The Asahi spherical charcoal has yet to be assessed in the test circuit but from the appearance of this charcoal (fig. 8, 9), similar results might be anticipated.

Apart from the Mitsubishi charcoal and the agarose beads, the fall in leucocytes was similar for the various uncoated and coated adsorbents. In contrast, the fall in platelets varied considerably. Albumin coating of Y56 resin (table II) showed that the fall in platelet level could be decreased using a solution of 1.0 g HSA/100 ml, with greater solution concentrations giving no further reduction in the fall. Albumin coating of Y56 had no apparent influence on the fall in leucocyte level. On the basis of these findings, it is suggested that the fall in platelet level and the fall in leucocyte level are caused by different mechanisms.

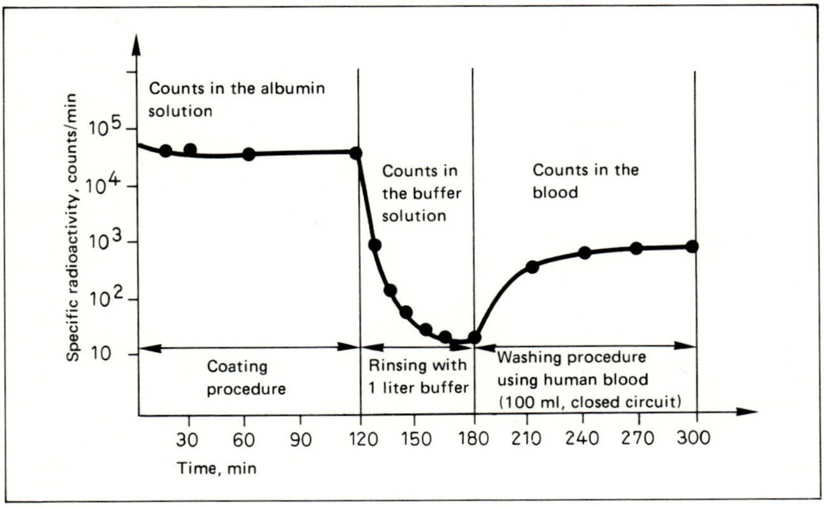

Fig. 10. Specific activity of rinsing solution and blood after albumin coating of Y56 resin.

The results of the fibrinogen adsorption (table III) demonstrate that the adsorption rate of fibrinogen correlates with the decrease in platelet drop obtained with coated and uncoated hemoadsorbents. Therefore, measurement of fibrinogen adsorption appears a valid test for blood compatibility.

The studies of adsorbent efficiency based on vitamin B_{12} clearance and the adsorption of drugs indicate that the spherical, activated charcoals are the most efficient. The studies also point out the marked decrease in efficiency resulting from excessive polymer coating.

The assessment of the various charcoals suggests that consideration should be given to the possibility of using uncoated spherical charcoal in certain clinical situations. If polymer coating of charcoal is adopted, the coating should be as thin as possible. Finally, there are advantages in using an ultrathin polymer coating in combination with an albumin coating, an approach which has been applied successfully by *Chang* [2].

Regarding the clinical use of Y56 resin in combination with albumin, it was of interest to assess the desorption of albumin. The desorption was investigated for a coating of 2% HSA using heparinized fresh blood. From figures 10 and 11, the desorption of albumin can be calculated to be about 5% of the adsorbed protein. Taking into account the results shown in figure 1, the conclusion drawn is that for the clinical use of resin Y56, an albumin coating obtained with a solution of 1–2 g HSA/100 ml appears suitable and that it is not necessary to extend the coating time beyond 30 min.

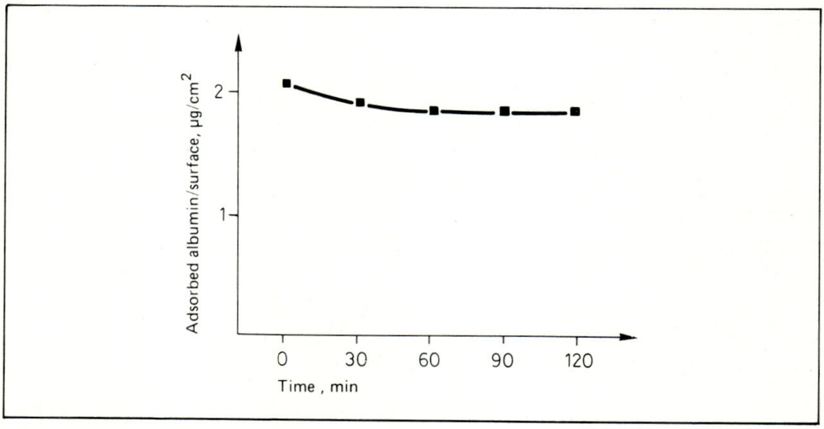

Fig. 11. Effect on the albumin coating of Y56 resin of washing with human blood.

This assessment has demonstrated that important information can be obtained from in vitro test procedures and that these procedures can be used to evaluate hemoadsorbents and to promote the development of improved hemoadsorbents for clinical application.

Summary

An in vitro assessment has been made of the blood compatibility and efficiency of different charcoal and resin hemoadsorbents. The charcoals vary in source, shape, size, nature and amount of polymer coating. The resins are the macroreticular adsorbents XAD-4 and Y56 and a carbonized resin. The effect on Y56 of albumin coating has been studied. The assessment has demonstrated that a reduction in platelet drop is accompanied by a decrease in the adsorption of fibrinogen. The results confirm the potential advantages of spherical charcoal and that coating with an ultrathin layer of polymer or with albumin does not seriously reduce efficiency. For Y56 resin, treatment with an albumin solution of 1–2 g/100 ml appears to be a suitable procedure if clinical use is considered.

References

1 Brunner, G.; Holloway, C.J.; Lösgen, H.: The application of immobilized enzymes in an artificial liver support system. Artificial Organs *3:* 27 (1979).

2 Chang, T.M.S.: Protective effects of microencapsulation (coating) on platelet depletion and particulate embolism in the clinical applications of charcoal haemoperfusion; in Kenedi, Courtney, Gaylor, Gilchrist, Artificial organs, p. 164 (Macmillan, London 1977).

3 Chang, T.M.S.: Assessment of clinical trials of charcoal hemoperfusion in uremic patients. Clin. Nephrol. *11:* 111 (1979).

4 Courtney, J.M.; Gaylor, J.D.S.; Maini, R.; Park, G.B.; Smith, E.S.: Strathclyde approach towards artificial kidney, artificial liver and detoxification; in Chang, Artificial kidney, artificial liver, and artificial cells; p. 225 (Plenum Press, New York 1978).

5 Falkenhagen, D.; Holtz, M.; Schmidt, R.; Gottschall, S.; Klinkmann, H.: In vitro und in vivo Untersuchungen mit Cellulose-Acetat umhüllten Aktivkohlen. II. Donausymposium für Nephrologie, p. 214 (Bindernagel, Friedberg 1978).

6 Falkenhagen, D.; Esther, G.; Ahrenholz, P.; Holtz, M.; Schmitt, E.; Klinkmann, H.: Blood compatibility and efficiency of different hemoadsorbents. Proc. Eur. Soc. Artif. Organs *7:* 137 (1980).

7 Gelfand, M.C.; Winchester, J.F.: Hemoperfusion uremia: results and future prospects; in Sideman, Chang, Hemoperfusion: kidney and liver support and detoxification, p. 231 (Hemisphere, Washington 1980).

8 Gurland, H.J.; Castro, L.A.; Hillebrand, G.; Schmidt, B.: Sorbent membranes and their medical applications; in Sideman, Chang, Hemoperfusion: kidney and liver support and detoxification, p. 105 (Hemisphere, Washington 1980).

9 Holloway, C.J.; Harstick, K.; Brunner, G.: Agarose-encapsulated adsorbents. Int. J. artif. Organs *2:* 81 (1979).

10 Klinkmann, H.; Falkenhagen, D.; Courtney, J.M.: Blood purification by haemoperfusion. Int. J. artif. Organs *2:* 296 (1979).

11 Rawer, R.; Leber, H.W.: Selektive Hämoperfusion. Medsche Welt, Stuttg. *29:* 1449 (1978).

12 Ryan, C.J.; Courtney, J.M.; Klinkmann, H.: Haematological changes induced by uncoated and coated charcoal in the rat. 15th Congr. Eur. Soc. Surgical Research (1980).

13 Shaldon, S.; Beau, M.C.; Claret, G.; Deschodt, G.; Mion, H.; Oules, R.; Ramperez, P.; Mion, C.: Sorbent regeneration of ultrafiltrate as a long-term treatment of end-stage renal failure. Artificial Organs *2:* 343 (1978).

14 Silk, D.B.A.; Williams, R.: Experiences in the treatment of fulminant hepatic failure by conservative therapy, charcoal haemoperfusion and polyacrylonitrile haemodialysis. Int. J. artif. Organs *1:* 29 (1978).

D. Falkenhagen, MD, Department of Medicine, Wilhelm Pieck University, Rostock (GDR)

Contr. Nephrol., vol. 29, pp. 34–52 (Karger, Basel 1982)

Reflections on the Role of Carbon Haemoadsorption in Therapeutic Medicine

T. Gilchrist

Bioengineering Unit, University of Strathclyde, Glasgow, Scotland

Introduction

Haemoperfusion studies at the University of Strathclyde were initiated during the early seventies very much under the influence of the earlier pioneering work of *Yatzidis* [60] and the ongoing clinical work being carried out by *Chang* [11–14] in Montreal. In Scotland our studies have included adsorbent selection [10, 23, 34], the synthesis and evaluation of novel polymer coatings [18, 19, 21, 22] and the development of a coating technique [20, 29]. In joint collaboration with the Tenovus Kidney Diseases Research Unit, Glasgow Royal Infirmary, a pre-clinical evaluation of haemoperfusion in acute poisoning and uraemia including studies of induced haemostatic changes has been carried out [32, 33, 50, 51, 55, 57–59]. Recently an additional technique has been developed which permits repeated haemoperfusion of the rat in an unrestrained and conscious state to allow studies covering various aspects of haemoperfusion to be carried out [45, 46]. A principal result of our work has been the recommendation of Norit RBX-1 extruded carbon for haemoperfusion [28].

Strathclyde coated carbon was first used clinically in 1973 as a treatment for acute drug intoxications [36] and thereafter has been evaluated for a wide range of drugs as well as for the treatment of uraemia and hepatic failure [27]. This led on to the commercial development of the Gambro Adsorba device still based on Norit RBX-1 activated carbon using cellulosic coating. Our clinical collaborators have continued to evaluate the role of carbon haemoadsorption in therapeutic medicine using the Adsorba 300 C [37–40] and also the Haemocol device [52, 54, 56, 59].

Selection of Activated Carbon

This was carried out in conjunction with Norit-Clydesdale [10] and was mainly concerned with the physical structure and strength of the activated carbons required for haemoperfusion purposes. The Norit RBX-1 which was finally selected for this medical use is a cylindrically shaped granular carbon produced by extruding previously carbonised powdered peat coke, with binder, followed by the carbonisation of the binder and then steam activation. Any large macropores present in the original carbonised material have been destroyed by grinding and so the largest pores in an extruded carbon are the interparticle interstices between the carbon particles. This means that it is possible to control the upper limit of the macropore structure and this is an important factor in this present application. The extruded granules are 2.3 mm in length with a diameter of 1 mm, which is sufficiently small to minimise wall effects in the perfusion column and to give a reasonable rate of adsorption without causing an excessive pressure differential across the device.

The mechanical strength of carbon is also important in this application because any particles which break off pass directly into the blood stream and cause embolic problems. With any range of steam-activated carbons, the mechanical strength decreases as the adsorptive properties increase. The reason for this is that the steam activation process depends upon a controlled steam/carbon reaction at a temperature of 800–1,000 °C. The reaction occurs at the carbon surface within the pore structure, thus developing the porosity by removing carbon from the pore walls which obviously decreases its strength. Accordingly a Norit extruded carbon of good abrasive resistance was selected with a surface area of 850 m^2/g. The acid-washed form is chosen as there are less inorganic impurities. The total surface area is determined by the BET method of benzene vapour adsorption and includes the micropore structure ($<$10 Å in diameter), the transitional pores and macropores ($>$2,000 Å). Using mercury porosimetry methods [9] the pore size distribution can be determined and this gives an area for the macropores of 0.8 m^2/g down to a pore radius of 2,000 Å. This represents the surface available to accept a polymer coating [10, 17, 48] leaving the much larger area of micropores freely available for the adsorption process.

Polymer Coatings for Norit RBX-1

The Strathclyde University Bioengineering Unit has been involved for many years in the synthesis and evaluation of membrane films for use in blood purification systems. *Courtney* [17] and *Courtney* et al. [21] concluded that there could be considerable advantages to be gained by using copolymer systems to form such membranes if one monomer component contributed to film strength and the other to sensitivity or surface reactivity. To date three acrylic copolymers have been evaluated as adsorbent coatings. The first is based on a copolymer of acrylic acid and n-butyl methacrylate [18] where the methacrylate constituent determines the mechanical characteristics of the membrane film and the acrylic acid gives rise to a water-sensitive charged membrane species. This copolymer can be used to membrane coat adsorbents or else it can be modified chemically to alter the surface charge and water sensitivity by reaction with ethylene oxide gas. The product of this reaction is a highly hydrophilic hydroxyethylacrylate polymer. The second is a copolymer of acrylonitrile (AN) and dimethylaminoethylmethacrylate (DMAEMA). Self-polymerisation of AN gives a highly stable polyacrylonitrile and therefore imparts strength to the copolymer whereas DMAEMA is the functional species in the sense that the cationic property arising from the tertiary amino group is retained after polymerisation. On self-polymerisation DMAEMA gives rise to a water-soluble material, but when blended into a copolymer with AN it forms water-sensitive cationic films which can be prepared by solvent casting procedures.

This copolymer membrane can be used as an adsorbent coating or additionally like the previous material it can be modified to alter the surface charge and water sensitivity. Here the reaction of ethylene oxide gas with the tertiary amino groups leads to the production of hydroxyethyl primary alcohol groups and also causes a structural change which produces a cyclised ladder polymer. The water sensitivity depends on the modification time and temperature.

The unmodified AN-DMAEMA membrane being cationic exhibits an affinity for the ionic attachment of heparin and studies [30, 31] have demonstrated that in 7 min the unmodified membranes can take up 17 times as much heparin as do the ethylene oxide-modified membranes. These latter membranes are no longer cationic and heparin is readily washed off their surfaces. This contrasts with the chemical binding of heparin to unmodified AN-DMAEMA surfaces where leaching rates at 70 h are less than 1.0%.

The third encapsulating material for carbon granules is a copolymer of DMAEMA and methylmethacrylate in the proportion 50:50 where once again the aminoester of methacrylic acid confers water sensitivity and cationic properties [21].

Polymer Coating of Norit RBX-1

These three copolymer systems have been used for coatings around the perfusion grade-activated carbon. In the Strathclyde coating process, washed and dried carbon particles are allowed to roll in an inclined, rotating vessel. The rotation causes the carbon particles to become positively charged. A wave pattern is assumed by the particles during rotation and a controlled mix is achieved while

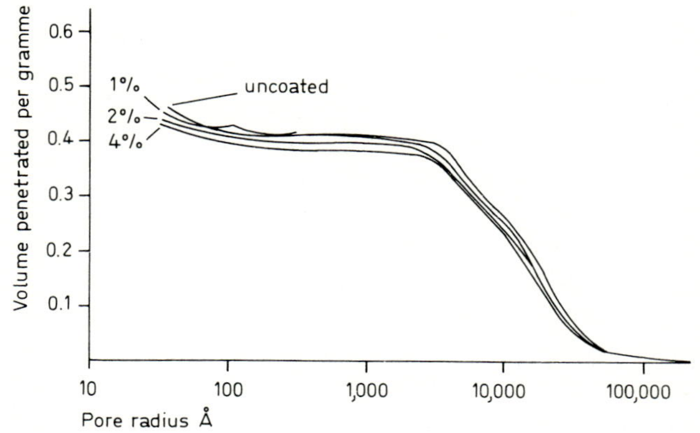

Fig. 1. Cumulative pore volume distribution of coated and uncoated Norit RBX-1.

contact between the granules is hindered by electrostatic repulsion. The polymer, dissolved in solvent, is added to the rotating vessel.

Rotation is continued until free flowing, non-adhering coated particles are obtained and the solvent adsorbed into or evaporated from the carbon. Thermal treatment of the particles prior to and following the coating process is selected in accordance with the boiling point of the solvent in use and ensures that the minimum amount of solvent remains adsorbed on completion of the process. In order to determine the areas of the carbon which were coated with the polymer, the cumulative pore size distributions of a series of coated carbons were determined using low and high pressure mercury porosimetry [10]. As the curves (fig. 1) are parallel below 2,000 Å it would suggest that most of the polymer is located in the macropore region (>2,000 Å). Considering the average molecular weight of these copolymers (e.g. the acrylic acid copolymer is approximately 80,000 MW), it is undeed unlikely that they can penetrate beyond the macropores. If it is assumed that only this region is coated with polymer then one can offer an estimate of the membrane thickness based on the macropore surface area of 0.8 m^2/g and the coating weight. For coating weights of 1–4% this gives a thickness variation from 125–500 Å which is approximately a hundred times less than that of a normal dialysis membrane and the rate of diffusion across the membrane coating will be very much greater. The effective surface area available for adsorption will approximate to 80 m^2 per 100 g of activated carbon charge.

Animal Studies

Several series of animal experiments have been carried out to evaluate the effectiveness of the Strathclyde coated Norit RBX-1 in acute poisoning induced by salicylates, paracetamol [50, 51] and paraquat [32, 33] and in uraemia and liver failure [1–3]. In one dog series, *Winchester* et al. [50, 51] studied the pharmacokinetics of paracetamol elimination by haemoperfusion. A simple mathematical model was developed to calculate in vivo clearance data. This demonstrated that both in vivo paracetamol clearance and elimination rates are increased by haemoadsorption. Previous drug elimination and drug distribution must be taken into consideration otherwise calculations can overestimate by approximately twofold the efficiency of haemoperfusion. Nevertheless, paracetamol elimination half-time was significantly decreased.

Working in the very difficult area of experimental hepatic coma, *Abouna* et al. [1–3] evolved several dog models for evaluating artificial hepatic support techniques. One satisfactory model can be produced by temporary ischaemia of the liver induced by end-to-side portacaval anastomosis, followed 24 h later by occlusion of the common hepatic and gastroduodenal arteries for a period of 1 h. This model complies with many important criteria. These include: that the liver injury produced be extensive, uniform and very rapid; that this be reproducible; that it be potentially reversible; that it results in hepatic coma with a very high mortality rate and that the animal survives in a fairly stable haemodynamic status long enough for the institution and evaluation of therapy.

Two investigations have been undertaken, the first using 100-g cartridges of Norit RBX-1 coated with AN-DMAEMA copolymer and the second using 120 g of the same carbon coated with cellulosic polymer. In the first study, 8 animals were treated by 3-hour haemoperfusions 4–6 h after completion of surgery and although several of the treated animals survived appreciably longer than the untreated controls, others died of bleeding due to the induced hepatic failure, overheparinisation and blood trauma induced by the perfusion.

The second study (table I) involving 21 animals included resin haemoperfusion (Amberlite XAD-4) for direct comparison and 2-hour haemoperfusions were carried out 5–6 h after induction of hepatic necrosis. Definite clinical improvement was observed in 4 animals treated by carbon haemoperfusion, but only in 2 animals receiving resin perfusion. From table I it can be seen that there is no difference in the recovery rate among the three groups, but survival following charcoal perfusion was significantly longer than that following resin treatment.

The tentative conclusions from these findings and observations are as follows: (1) Haemoperfusion with activated carbon and Amberlite resin XAD-4 does sometimes produce a marked clinical improvement in animals with experimental hepatic failure. (2) Such improvement is temporary and one haemoper-

Table I. Liver haemoperfusion: animal survival

Group	Animals h	Number recovered	Death from coma, %	Mean survival h	Range of survival, h
1 (control)	9	2	77.7	27.5 ± 12.0	16–40
2 (charcoal)	6	2	66.6	46.25 ± 10.6	20–72
3 (resin)	6	2	66.6	18.65 ± 4.2	7–26

fusion does not seem to alter the mortality rate from hepatic failure. (3) Haemoperfusion with activated charcoal is superior to resin perfusion, both in the clinical results and in the seriousness of complications. (4) The biochemical changes associated with charcoal and with resin haemoperfusion do not appear either specific or consistent. Although marked adsorption of free fatty acids and octopamine was seen following these perfusions, such changes were not observed in those amino acids or other compounds which are generally thought to contribute to the neurological manifestations of hepatic coma. (5) Haemoperfusion with either charcoal or Amberlite resin can only have a very limited role in the treatment of hepatic coma and in our opinion these techniques by themselves can do little to alter the many potentially lethal systemic and metabolic manifestations of the syndrome of hepatic failure which are often the cause of death in this condition.

Our choice of animal species has been varied and while dog studies have predominated we have more recently developed a technique which permits repeated haemoperfusion of the rat in an unrestrained and conscious state [45, 46]. This involves a surgical procedure for implantation of indwelling carotid arterial and jugulo-venous cannulae. Teflon tubing is used and the cannulae are tunnelled subcutaneously over each shoulder and brought out through the dorsal surface midway between the scapulae. They are passed through a harness consisting of flexible Silastic tubing connected to a shouldered (cuffed) end polypropylene tube. The animals are placed in a specially designed haemoperfusion cage and both the arterial and the venous cannulae are attached to a free rotating disc situated at the top of the cage. A heparin block is maintained to prevent clotting of the lines. Haemoperfusion can be performed in both the unrestrained and unanaesthetised state, using columns charged with 1.4 g activated carbon at a flow rate of 1 ml/min over periods of up to 4 h each on 4 consecutive days. This is equivalent to a 400-gramme charge for a 70-kg male and to a comparable blood flow rate of 200 ml/min.

The small extracorporeal volume of 2.5–2.75 ml permits priming with heparinised saline, thus eliminating the possible effects of using donor blood or plasma and also leads to minimal blood loss after each perfusion. Studies in the normal rat demonstrated minimal long-term metabolic and biochemical changes associated with repeated haemoperfusion and a further study following partial hepatectomy has shown that haemoperfusion over the activated carbon does not influence the capability of the liver to regenerate following hepatic injury and that liver mass function and fat content consequent upon partial hepatectomy are also not influenced.

Blood Compatibility

All procedures involving the circulation of blood through extracorporeal devices lead inevitably to blood-foreign surface interactions. Species variations do occur especially in the response of the cellular elements, but the trends made evident in animal experiments can anticipate the likely human response.

Thrombocytopenia is a recurring feature of carbon haemoperfusion in both man and animals, but is not always a problem [15, 38]. Observed falls of up to 50–60% have been recorded when patients were subjected to this treatment [5, 24, 26, 47]. Similar falls have been observed during our animal studies [1, 3, 32, 45] with the most profound drops occurring in animals with liver failure where platelet function is deeply distrubed by the clinical status itself. Rebound does take place and *Abouna* et al. [1, 3] showed a response in dogs from an initial fall of up to 50% by the end of the perfusion, returning to greater than 75% of the initial pre-perfusion values within 24 h after completion of the treatment. Using the rat model, *Ryan* et al. [45] observed a response in animals subjected to haemoperfusion of up to 4 h duration over Norit RBX-1 coated with AN-DMAEMA, where the post-perfusion levels of 17% returned to within normal levels by the next perfusion period 20 h later. Uncoated carbon was responsible for platelet depletion levels after perfusion of 40–50%. By contrast, animals perfused through an empty column showed only a slight reduction in platelet count with values still remaining within normal levels.

Minor changes in erythrocyte levels occurring during perfusion in animals and humans have been found to disappear within 24 h. Sequestration leucopenia also occurs, although the predominant feature is the passage of blood through the extracorporeal circuit rather than any influence of the adsorbent, and normal leucocyte levels are achieved a few hours after perfusion.

In an attempt to simulate clinical haemoperfusion while assessing the blood compatibility of adsorbents and their coatings, we have established a technique for the recirculation of healthy human blood or platelet-rich plasma through a miniature column containing the adsorbent [53, 57, 58].

This test system was used to evaluate the AN-DMAEMA copolymer-coated Norit RBX-1 carbon in vitro over 2-hour perfusions. We have shown that in heparinised blood the platelet depletion was only 15% compared with a value of

90% depletion with uncoated carbon. Citrated blood resulted in equivalent values (20%) for platelet falls with either coated or uncoated carbons. Coagulation factors II, V, IX, X and XII in the blood were reduced following either coated or uncoated carbon perfusion, but associated changes in coagulation tests (KCCT, PTT etc.) only occurred with the uncoated carbon.

Replacement of the whole blood with heparinised platelet-rich plasma in the perfusion circuit resulted in small changes in platelet levels after passage through coated or uncoated carbon. It would seem from this study that heparinised human blood when perfused over activated carbon will exhibit less platelet depletion and reduced changes in coagulation factors if the carbon has a copolymer coating. Since the red cell-free perfusion produced only small falls in platelets, it would appear that red cell adenosine diphosphate may play a crucial role in producing platelet aggregation/adhesion to the artificial surfaces in direct contact with blood during haemoperfusion.

Clinical Experience

Strathclyde Acrylic Polymer Coatings

Clinical use of Norit RBX-1-extruded carbon for blood detoxification commenced early in 1975 when *Gilchrist* et al. [27] and *Martin* et al. [36] haemoperfused patients with chronic uraemia and overdosages of Doriden (glutethimide), paracetamol and tricyclic antidepressants and also perfused a patient in hepatic failure (tables II, III). All but one of these treatments utilized a dialyser in series with the carbon column. The very first devices used did give rise to rigors in 3 patients, but subsequently no adverse physical effects were observed during treatments. Variations in pressure were similar to those seen in standard haemodialysis and platelet loss was minimal. The success in the treatment of 1 case of glutethimide poisoning by this means prompted its evaluation in a further 5 patients (table IV). These were all severely poisoned in grade IV coma with blood levels of glutethimide ranging from 180 to 350 μmol/l. Blood levels in excess of 138 μmol/l carry associated mortality between 50 and 60% from cerebral oedema, pulmonary oedema and hypotension. This is considered to be linked to a metabolite of glutethimide which interfaces with steroid synthesis. Clearance of the column (100-gramme charge) and dialyser together ranged from 83 to 120 ml/min and all 5 patients recovered.

Cellulosic Polymer Coatings.

The first-generation acrylic copolymer-based devices were exchanged for the commercially produced Adsorba 300 C columns charged with 300-gramme Norit RBX-1 carbon granules carrying a cellulosic coating. Clinical evaluation [37, 38] was undertaken in acute poisoning (amylo barbitone, pentobarbitone and paraquat) and in uraemia. The clearances demonstrated for short-acting barbiturates

Table II. Clinical trials 1973 – Strathclyde devices

Patient	Diagnosis	Charge, g	Duration, h	Q_b, ml/min	Platelets $\frac{post}{pre} \times 10^3$
1	Paracetamol	400	1	200	100/210
2	Uraemia	100	1	100	116/119
3	Uraemia	100	1.25	100	112/85
4	Uraemia	400	2	200	305/355
5	Tofranil	200	2	136	150/190
6	Doriden	100	2	206	160/220

Table III. Clinical trials 1974 – Strathclyde devices

Patient	Diagnosis	Heparin	Charge g	Duration h	Q_b, ml/min	Platelets $\frac{post}{pre} \times 10^3$
1	Uraemia	7,500	100	2	176	112/160
2	Uraemia	7,500	200	20 min	200	180/260
3	Uraemia	7,500	100	1	200	465/510
4	Uraemia	7,500	100	1	200	275/350
5	Uraemia	7,500	100	15 min	200	111/450
6	Uraemia	12,000	100	2	176	200/280
7	Uraemia	10,000	100	20 min	176	188/225
8	Uraemia	7,500	150	1	176	120/325
9	Uraemia	7,500	150	1	176	152/280

Table IV. Severe glutethimide poisoning: combined hemodialysis/hemoperfusion

Patient	Glutethimide blood levels, μmol/l			
	clearance ml/min	before treatment	after 2 h	fully conscious after
1	66 column only	225.4	101.2	2 h
2	120 column and dialysis	188.6	115.0	10 h
3	104 column and dialysis	225.4	96.6	11 h
4	84 column and dialysis	345.0	220.8	30 h
5	–	289.8	184.0	24 h

Table V. Short-acting barbiturate poisoning

Patient	Blood flow ml/min	Perfusion time min	Clearance ml/min	Pre-drug levels mg/l	Post-drug levels mg/l
1	240	90	38	36	21
2	250	30	30	28	18
3	218	20	43	38	19
	240	40	10		
	240	60	21		
	240	90	10		

Amylobarbitone removal rate up to 375 mg/h; 300 g carbon.

Table VI. Haemoperfusion in ESRD using Adsorba 300 C devices: mean data for creatinine and uric acid clearance

Charge	300 g Norit RBX-1
Coating	3–5 μm Cellulose
Clearance	
Creatinine	101–179 ml/min at Q_b 200–400
Uric acid	105–127 ml/min at Q_b 200–400
Platelets post-perfusion	90–96%

Table VII. Haemoperfusion in ESRD: patient data over 2-month period

Creatinine, μmol/l		Uric acid, mmol/l	
pre-perfusion	post-perfusion	pre-perfusion	post-perfusion
940	550	0.53	0.28
960	790	0.54	0.43
1,030	790	0.56	0.40
1,040	880	0.51	0.42
950	510	0.51	0.27
940	490	0.56	0.26
840	420	0.50	0.23

(table V) were much superior to those recorded for haemodialysis and peritoneal dialysis with removal rates of up to 375 mg/h.

Haemoperfusion was also carried out in 4 end-stage uraemics who were well and stable on regular dialysis. No adverse reactions to the produre were observed. Perfusion times ranged from 2 to 3.5 h with a blood flow rate of 240–280 ml/min. The platelet changes were insignificant as a results of the perfusions and creatinine clearance ranged from 101 to 179 ml/min, uric acid ranged from 105 to 127 ml/min, the fall in blood levels amounting to about 50% of the pre-perfusion concentration in most cases. Mean data for concentration changes of creatinine, uric acid and the mean platelet changes are documented in table VI. 1 patient, a 20-year-old male on regular home dialysis, was treated by haemoperfusion on ten occasions alternating with haemodialysis over a 2-month period (table VII). Again there was no significant platelet abnormality during or after any of the haemoperfusions. These 2-hour treatments in end-stage renal disease, when alternated with haemodialysis in the short term on a repeated basis, demonstrate satisfactory symptomatic and biochemical control of the uraemic state.

Uraemic Pericarditis

Uraemic pericarditis is a fibrino-haemorrhagic form of inflammation of the pericardial sac that develops in patients with renal faulure. It was first described in 1836 by *Bright* [7]. Pericarditis develops in 50% of non-dialysed patients who have severe renal failure [49]. Despite the advent of what is considered adequate dialysis the overall incidence is thought to be between 4 and 18% [6, 16, 35, 41]. The pathogenesis and course remains poorly understood and there may well be two forms occurring in the uraemic, the first form in those who have never been dialysed and the second form in dialysed patients, which has been described as 'dialysis-associated pericarditis'. An infective cause is rarely identified and there is a poor correlation with measurable biochemical parameters including middle molecules in dialysed patients. No relationship to the length of time on dialysis has been established. There may be multiple causative factors.

Treatment regimes aimed at curing uraemic pericarditis include daily or alternate-day dialysis, ultrafiltration and intensified haemodialysis [4] and the use of intrapericardial corticosteroids [8]. The total duration of the illness has ranged from 1 to 22 weeks (mean 6.4 weeks). The mortality has ranged from 12 to 90%, the high mortality occurring in 'dialysis-associated' pericarditis with cardiac tamponade [42]. In relation to the etiology, and the possible correlation of fibrinous pericarditis with plasma fibrinolytic activity, a group of patients who developed pericarditis on dialysis was studied [16]. The pericarditis was found to be associated with reduced plasma fibrinolytic activity and it was suggested that this may be a pathogenic factor in the development of fibrinous pericarditis.

Assessing the efficacy of therapy remains purely clinical, relying on the duration of the illness, mortality of whether the patient ultimately requires

Table VIII. Pericarditis: patient data

Patient	Age	Time on dialysis prior to pericarditis, months	Pre-dialysis blood urea, mm/l		
			before illness	at onset	after resolution
1	48	60	25	31	21.5
2	26	1	37	31.8	28
3	51	40	36	45	30
4	58	14	31	46	39.7
5	34	15	28.7	42.8	34.7
6	46	6	25.5	57	31.7
7	45	19	35	52	34.6
8	60	0		85	34
9	58	0		35.5	31.2
10	48	0		34	25.2
11	58	0		39.8	25.8
12	39	0		52	27.1
13	35	0		58	25.7

pericardictomy. This is generally recommended for pericardial effusion which has not diminished after 10–14 days of conservative treatment. In the first clinical trials of carbon haemoperfusion in uraemia, *Yatzidis* [60] treated one patient with uraemic pericarditis and observed resolution of signs and symptoms within 12 h.

Cellulose-coated carbon haemoperfusion was incorporated into the treatment regime of 9 patients with uraemic pericarditis in order to assess whether the duration of the illness could be reduced. The study was undertaken in view of the report of *Yatzidis* [60] and subsequent to observing the response of one patient whose pericarditis persisted after a regime of intensified dialysis until the introduction of haemoperfusion. Signs and symptoms of pericarditis resolved rapidly after four perfusions. This treatment regime was compared retrospectively with 4 patients who had not received carbon haemoperfusion but simply dialysis therapy. Haemodialysis was undertaken in all patients for 3–3.5 h using a 1.5-m^2 coil device (Ultraflow 100) or a 0.92-m^2 capillary plate dialyser (Holtzenbein). Patients receiving haemoperfusion treatment were perfused for 3 h at a blood flow rate of 200–250 ml/min through a column of cellulose-coated activated carbon.

The patient data before and after pericarditis, the treatment schedules and duration of pericarditis are documented in tables VIII and IX. 7 patients had been maintained on regular dialysis for periods ranging from 1 month to 60 months prior to the onset of pericarditis. 6 patients developed pericarditis while awaiting a place on the dialysis programme. The 4 cases that were treated by

Table IX. Pericarditis: treatment and duration

Patient	Treatment	Treatments h	Duration of illness days
1	HD/PD/P	35	61
2	HD	15	28
3	HD/PD/P	14	32
4	HD/PD	19	30
5	HD/HP (4)	30	33
6	HD/HP (3)	4	6
7	HD/HP (3)	11	18
8	HD/PD/HP (5)	10	10
9	HD/PD/HP (3)	8	11
10	HD/PD/HP (5)	8	9
11	HD/HP (5)	14	20
12	HD/PD/HP (3)	10	12
13	HD/PD/HP (3)	8	12

HD = haemodialysis; P = pericardiectomy; PD = peritoneal dialysis; HP = carbon haemoperfusion.

dialysis alone required from 14 to 35 treatments and the duration of the illness ranged from 28 to 51 days. 2 of these patients required pericardectomy for tamponade in one and chronic constriction in the other case. Patient 5 was treated by haemodialysis alone on 20 occasions over a period of 23 days without resolution. Cellulose-coated carbon haemoperfusion was introduced into the schedule on four occasions over the following 10 days and the pericarditis resolved within 36 h of the last haemoperfusion. 8 patients were treated with a combination of dialysis and cellulose-coated carbon haemoperfusion from the onset of the illness, they required 4–14 treatments, the duration of the illness ranged from 6 to 20 days. No patient died during the phase of active pericarditis.

The Effects of Carbon Haemoperfusion on Fibrinolysis

Fibrinolytic activity is abnormal in acute and chronic renal failure [16]. Regular haemodialysis patients have been shown to have both normal and abnormal fibrinolytic activity between treatments and the development of uraemic pericarditis is associated with reduced fibrinolytic activity. With a view to assessing the efficacy of various treatment regimes in correcting abnormalities in fibrinolysis, an evaluation of the acute effects of dialysis and haemoperfusion was undertaken [39].

Table X. Euglobulin clot lysis time (min): carbon haemoperfusion/haemodialysis paired studies

Carbon haemoperfusion			Haemodialysis		
before	after 2 h	after 3 h	before	after 2 h	after 3 h
258	78		258	138	
342	60		324	132	
126	168		144	132	144
204	30	72	204	204	
216	36		222	186	208
168	42		180	184	
258	54		234	90	
336	36	168	324	288	324
378	180		360	240	
396	198	268	402	348	

The euglobulin clot lysis time (ECLT) was assessed as a measure of fibrinolytic activity using citrated plasma. Analyses were undertaken before, during and after treatment by haemodialysis (Holtzenbein, Gambro Lundia) cellulose-coated carbon haemoperfusion (Adsorba 300 C), and peritoneal dialysis. A series of normal control analyses were also undertaken. Haemodialysis and haemoperfusion was undertaken for 2 or 3 h at blood flow rates of 200–250 ml/min. 41 studies were made in 10 uraemic patients, comprising 24 studies in 5 patients with end-stage renal failure established on regular dialysis (3–3.5 h thrice weekly). 12 studies were carried out in 3 patients with acute renal failure. Five studies were undertaken in 2 patients with chronic renal failure receiving intermittent peritoneal dialysis therapy.

The mean ECLT in healthy volunteer controls was 149 min. The results of 36 studies undertaken in 8 patients with acute and chronic renal failure before and after haemodialysis and cellulose-coated carbon haemoperfusion are illustrated in table X. In 5 end-stage uraemics on regular dialysis 24 studies were undertaken comparing haemodialysis and cellulose-coated carbon haemoperfusion. The mean pre-dialysis ECLT was 239 min. The mean ECLT at 2 h was 168 min and at 3 h was 220 min. The mean pre-haemoperfusion ECLT was 219 min. The mean ECLT at 2 h was 80 min and at 3 h was 168 min.

Ten paired studies documented in table X compare haemoperfusion and haemodialysis for similar pre-treatment ECLT values. The difference in ECLT (between haemoperfusion and haemodialysis) after 2 h therapy was statistically significant. With peritoneal dialysis there was no difference in fibrinogen levels before and after any of the treatment undertaken. Prolongation of ECLT in uraemia and particularly in uraemic pericarditis may have some pathological significance. In pericarditis, fibrin covers the pericardial surface and can lead to constrictive pericarditis. Small vessel coagulation is known to occur in uraemia and has been thought to be one factor in causing acute renal failure by means of glomerular thrombosis [43]. Accelerating fibrinolysis could be of value in uraemia and the effect of cellulose-coated carbon haemoperfusion and to a lesser extent haemodialysis would certainly explain some of the success observed in the management of uraemic pericarditis. The adsorption of $\alpha_2$globulins (an integral component of antifibrinolysins) might explain this effect and further study is required. A prophylactic role for cellulose-coated carbon haemoperfusion might be considered in end-stage uraemics who are found to have prolonged ECLT. In acute reversible renal failure similarly, the definition of a prolonged ECLT might suggest the use of a regime such as haemoperfusion in order to prevent thrombotic lesions which may result in structural glomerular change.

Conclusions

Many clinicians and bioengineers have been seeking to find a positive role for activated carbon haemoperfusion in therapeutic medicine. Its use has been widely explored in acute poisoning, uraemia and liver failure and because its mode of action in blood detoxification is somewhat different to dialysis, it has been considered as a possible treatment for chronic schizophrenia, psoriasis and rheumatism for example and in such outstanding uraemic problems as pruritus, pericarditis, neuropathy and pigmentation.

Acute Poisonings. We are well in agreement with views exposed by others working in this area [44] who have concluded that adsorbent haemoperfusion can produce high clearance rates for many induced intoxicants including the sedative hypnotics and analgesics which feature in so many acute poisoning episodes. There is no appreciable clinical toxicity and such treatment does lead to a rapid restoration of vital functions. Despite strong counter-arguments [25] against extracorporeal intervention in acute drug intoxication we believe that these beneficial clinical effects do justify haemoperfusion in deeply comatose patients.

Liver Failure. The present consensus of medical opinion [47] is that a life support device to counter hepatic encephalopathy is required which will act to prevent accumulation of high levels of water-soluble and protein-bound toxins in the blood. Existing technology has not yet supplied the answer. Activated carbon can presently be described as merely one component in a partially assembled system which awaits other active constituents.

Uraemia. Our work has shown in end-stage renal disease that a 2-hour haemoperfusion will reduce the concentrations of creatinine and uric acid by 50%. Used in the short term on a repeated basis, alternated with haemodialysis, carbon adsorption results in satisfactory symptomatic and biochemical control of the uraemic state. Nevertheless the dominant, essential role in this life support therapy is still provided by haemodialysis. Similar conclusions have been drawn by all other workers who have undertaken trials of carbon haemoperfusion in uraemia. An adsorbent-based therapy must await additional materials which will extend the partial detoxification role played by carbon. For the present the contribution of carbon appears limited to that of a temporary adjunct to dialysis for the more effective treatment of certain secondary complications such as pericarditis and pruritis, neuropathy and pigmentation.

Summary

The selection of Norit RBX-1-activated carbon granules for blood detoxification by haemoadsorption is outlined. Synthetic polymer membranes have been coated on to this carbon by a specially developed process and perfusion devices prepared from these materials have been evaluated in animal models of acute poisoning and liver failure. Clinical application of carbon haemoadsorption has been explored in acute poisoning, liver failure and uraemia. The experience to date would suggest that carbon will have to be augmented by other adsorbent species before life support systems based principally on haemoadsorption become a reality especially in the treatment of uraemia and in liver failure. A secondary role as a temporary adjunct to dialysis has been established for carbon haemoperfusion in the treatment of uraemic pericarditis and is under further investigation in the treatment of pruritis, pigmentation and neuropathy.

References

1 Abouna, G.M.; Gilchrist, T.; Pettit, J.E.; Boyd, N.D.; Todd, J.K.; Courtney, J.M.; Maini, R.: Haemoperfusion with activated charcoal in treatment of experimental acute hepatic failure; in Williams, Murray-Lyon, Artificial liver support, p. 180 (Pitman Medical, London 1975).

2 Abouna, G.M.; Barabas, A.Z.; Alexander, F.; Boyd, N.; Todd, J.K.; Kinniburgh, D.W.; Gilchrist, T.: Animal models of hepatic failure for evaluation of artificial liver support techniques; in Kenedi, Courtney, Gaylor, Gilchrist, Artificial organs, p. 351 (Macmillan, London 1977).

3 Abouna, G.M.; Barabas, A.Z.; Boyd, N.; Todd, J.K.; Alexander, F.; Kinniburgh, D.W.; Gilchrist, T.; Jonsson, E.: Resin and charcoal haemoperfusion in the treatment of hepatic coma; in Kenedi, Courtney, Gaylor, Gilchrist, Artificial organs, p. 363 (Macmillan, London 1977).

4 Ahmed, R.; Goldsmith, H.J.: A response of pericardial effusion to ultrafiltration and intensified haemodialysis. Dialysis Transplant. vol. no. 6, p. 12 (1977).

5 Amano, I.; Kano, H.; Takahira, H.; Yamamoto, Y.; Itoh, K.; Iwatsuki, S.; Maeda, K.; Ohta, K.: Hepatic assist system using bead type charcoal; in Chang, Artificial kidney, artificial liver and artificial cells, p. 89 (Plenum Press, New York 1978).

6 Bailey, G.L.; Hampers, C.L.; Hager, E.B.; Merrill, J.P.: Uraemic pericarditis. Clinical features and management. Circulation *38:* 582 (1968).

7 Bright, R.: Tabular view of the morbid appearance in 100 cases connected with albuminous urine. Guy's Hosp. Rep. *1:* 380 (1836).

8 Buselmeier, T.J.; Simmons, R.L.; Najarian, J.S.; Von Hartitzsch, B.; Bietzman, R.H.; Kjellstrand, C.M.: Intractable uraemic pericardial effusion. Proc. EDTA *10:* 289 (1973).

9 Cameron, A.; Stacy, W.O.: Pore size distribution in activated carbons. Chemy Ind. *9:* 222 (1960).

10 Cameron, A.; Courtney, J.M.; Gilchrist, T.; MacDowall, J.; Walker, J.M.: The selection and use of activated carbon to treat kidney diseases and drug overdose. Proc. 4th London Int. Carbon and Graphite Conf. (Pennard, London 1974).

11 Chang, T.M.S.: Semipermeable microcapsules. Science *146:* 524 (1964).

12 Chang, T.M.S.: Semipermeable aqueous microcapsules ('artificial cells'): with emphasis on experiments in an extracorporeal shunt system. Trans. Am. Soc. artif. internal Organs *12:* 13 (1966).

13 Chang, T.M.S.: Removal of endogenous and exogenous toxins by a microencapsulated adsorbent. Can. J. Physiol. Pharmacol. *47:* 1043 (1969).

14 Chang, T.M.S.: Artificial cells (Thomas, Springfield 1972).

15 Chang, T.M.S.: Protective effects of microencapsulation on platelet and particulate embolism in the clinical applications of charcoal haemoperfusion; in Kenedi, Courtney, Gaylor, Gilchrist, Artificial organs, p. 164 (Macmillan, London 1977).

16 Cochran, M.; Lawton, S.; Rowlands, M.M.: Fibrinous pericarditis and fibrinolysis in chronic dialysis patients. Clin. Nephrol. *11:* 23 (1979).

17 Courtney, J.M.: PhD thesis, University of Strathclyde (1969).

18 Courtney, J.M.; Gilchrist, T.; Walker, J.M.; Edwards, R.O.: A new coated adsorbent for blood perfusion. Dig. 10th Int. Conf. Med. Biol. Eng., p. 133 (1973).

19 Courtney, J.M.; Gilchrist, T.; Dunlop, E.H.: Coated adsorbent materials. US Patent 3, 983, 053, September 28 (1976).

20 Courtney, J.M.; Gilchrist, T.; Hood, R.G.; Townsend, W.B.: A novel method for preparing coated carbon granules. Proc. Eur. Soc. artif. Organs *2:* 210 (1976).

21 Courtney, J.M.; Fairweather, I.A.; Gilchrist, T.; Hood, R.G.; Park, G.B.; Smith, E.M.: The design of a polymer coating for activated carbon granules; in Kenedi, Courtney, Gaylor, Gilchrist, Artificial organs, p. 133 (Macmillan, London 1977).

22 Courtney, J.M.; Gaylor, J.D.S.; Maini, R.; Park, G.B.; Smith, E.M.: Strathclyde approach towards artificial kidney, artificial liver and detoxification; in Chang, Artificial kidney, artificial liver and artificial cells, p. 225 (Plenum Press, New York 1978).

23 Denti, E.; Walker, J.M.; Tessore, V.; Courtney, J.M.; Gilchrist, T.: New sorbent materials: vitreous carbon and carbon cloth. Cong. Italian Soc. of Nephrology, (Trieste 1978).

24 Dunea, G.; Kolff, W.J.: Clinical experiments and the Yatzidis charcoal artificial kidney. Trans. Am. Soc. artif. internal Organs *11:* 178 (1965).

25 Farrell, P.C.: Acute drug intoxication and extracorporeal intervention. J. Am. Soc. artif. internal Organs *3:* 39 (1980).

26 Gelfand, M.C.; Knepshield, J.H.; Cohan, S.; Ramirez, B.; Schreiner, G.E.: Treatment of hepatic coma with haemoperfusion through polyacrylamide hydrogel-coated charcoal. Kidney int. *10:* 239 (1976).

27 Gilchrist, T.; Johnsson, E.; Martin, A.M.; Naucler, L.; Cameron, A.; Courtney, J.M.: Development of the Strathclyde haemoperfusion system; in Williams, Murray-Lyon, Artificial liver support, p. 319 (Pitman Medical, London 1975).

28 Gilchrist, T.: Coated adsorbents in therapeutic medicine. Report (1974–77) to ACMR Study Group (Scottish Home and Health Department, 1978).

29 Hood, R.G.; Courtney, J.M.; Gilchrist, T.; Gaylor, J.D.S.: A method of coating granules. Br. Patent 1, 496, 330, December 30 (1977).

30 Lindsay, R.M.; Rourke, J.T.B.; Reid, B.D., Friesen, M.; Linton, A.L.; Courtney, J.M.; Gilchrist, T.: Platelets foreign-surfaces and heparin. Trans. Am. Soc. artif. internal Organs *12:* 292–295 (1976).

31 Lindsay, R.M.; Rourke, J.T.B.; Reid, B.D.; Linton, A.L.; Gilchrist, T.; Courtney, J.M.; Edwards, R.O.: The role of heparin on platelet retention by acrylonitrile copolymer dialysis membranes. J. Lab. clin. Med. *89:* 724 (1977).

32 Maini, R.; Winchester, J.F.: Removal of paraquat from blood by haemoperfusion over sorbent materials. Br. med. J. *iii:* 281 (1975).

33 Maini, R.; Courtney, J.M.; Gilchrist, T.; Winchester, J.F.; MacKay, J.M.: Paraquat removal by ion exchange haemoperfusion. Proc. Eur. Soc. artif. Organs *2:* 222 (1976).

34 Maini, R.: Haemoperfusion over ion exchange resins and polymeric adsorbents. Int. J. artif. Organs *1:* 196 (1978).

35 Marini, P.V.; Hull, A.R.: Uraemic pericarditis. A review of incidence and management. Kidney int., suppl. 2, p. 163 (1975).

36 Martin, A.M.; Mitchell, D.C.; Gibbins, J.K.; Devapal, D.; Trinder, P.: Charcoal haemoperfusion in the management of severe poisoning. Br. med. J. *i:* 392 (1975).

37 Martin, A.M., Gibbins, J.K.; Jonsson, E.; Trinder, P.: The clinical use of a carbon haemoperfusion column; in Kenedi, Courtney, Gaylor, Gilchrist, Artificial organs, p. 196 (Macmillan, London 1977).

38 Martin, A.M.; Gibbins, J.K.; Oduro, A.; Herbert, R.: Clinical experience with cellulose-coated carbon hemoperfusion; in Chang, Artificial kidney, artificial liver and artificial cells, p. 143 (Plenum Press, New York 1978).

39 Martin, A.M.; Gibbins, J.K.; Kimmett, J.; Rennie, F.: Haemodialysis and haemoperfusion in the treatment of uraemic pericarditis. Dialysis Transplant. *8:* 135 (1979).

40 Martin, A.M.; Gibbins, J.K.; Jones, T.; Smith, C.: Haemoperfusion and fibrinolysis. Trans. Am. Soc. artif. internal Organs (1980).

41 Mitchell, A.G.: Pericarditis during chronic haemodialysis therapy. Post-grad. med. J. *50:* 590, 741 (1974).

42 Pabico, R.C.; Freeman, R.B.: Pericarditis and myocardiopathy; in Massry, Sellars, Clinical aspects of uraemia and dialysis, vol. 4, p. 69 (Thomas, Springfield 1976).

43 Robson, J.S.; Clarkson, A.R.; MacDonald, M.K.; Fuster, V.; Cash, J.D.: Glomerular coagulations in acute ischaemic renal failure. Q. Il. Med. *39:* 156, 585 (1970).

44 Rosenbaun, J.L.: Poisonings; in Giordano, Sorbents and their clinical applications, chapter 19 (Academic Press, 1980).

45 Ryan, C.J.; Courtney, J.M.; Wood, C.B.; Hood, R.G.; Blumgart, J.H.: Activated charcoal haemoperfusion via an extracorporeal circuit in the unrestrained and unanaesthetised rat. Br. J. exp. Path. *60:* (1979).

46 Ryan, C.J.; Courtney, J.M.: Hemoperfusion in the rat: application to adsorbent evaluation; in Hemoperfusion: kidney and liver supports and detoxification (Hemisphere Publishing Corp., Washington, to be published).

47 Silk, D.B.A.; Williams, R.: Sorbents in hepatic failure; in Giordano, Sorbents and their clinical applications (Academic Press, 1980).

48 Tijssen, J.; Bantjes, A.; Van Doorn, A.W.J.; Feijen, J.; Van Dijk, B.; Vonk, C.R.; Dijkhuis, I.C.: A hemoperfusion column based on activated carbon granules coated with an ultrathin membrane of cellulose acetate. Artif. Organs *3:* 11 (1979).
49 Wacker, W.; Merrill, J.P.: Uraemic pericarditis in acute and chronic renal failure. J. Am. med. Ass. *156:* 746 (1954).
50 Winchester, J.F.; Tilstone, W.J.; Edwards, R.O.; Gilchrist, T.; Kennedy, A.C.: Hemoperfusion for enhanced drug elimination – a kinetic analysis in paracetamol poisoning. Trans. Am. Soc. artif. internal Organs *20:* 358 (1974).
51 Winchester, J.F.; Edwards, R.O.; Tilstone, W.J.; Woodcock, B.G.: Activated charcoal hemoperfusion and experimental acetaminophen poisoning. Toxicol. appl. Pharmacol. *31:* 120 (1975).
52 Winchester, J.F.; Apiliga, M.T.; MacKay, J.M.; Kennedy, A.C.: Haemodialysis with charcoal haemoperfusion. Proc. Eur Dialysis Transplant. Ass. *12:* 526 (1975).
53 Winchester, J.F.; MacKay, J.M.; Forbes, C.D.; Blackely, E.; Prentice, C.R.M.; Kennedy, A.C.; Harvey, B.; Gilchrist, T.: Haemostatic changes induced in vitro by activated charcoal haemoperfusion. Thromb. Diath. haemorrh. *34:* 587 (1975).
54 Winchester, J.F.; Apiliga, M.T.; Kennedy, A.C.: Short-term evaluation of charcoal hemoperfusion combined with dialysis in uremic patients. Kidney int. *10:* 315 (1976).
55 Winchester, J.F.: Comparison of charcoal hemoperfusion with hemodialysis. Dialysis Transplant. *6:* 46 (1977).
56 Winchester, J.F.: Clinical application of haemoperfusion in uraemia; in Kenedi, Cortney, Gaylor, Gilchrist, Artificial organs, p. 188 (Macmillan Press, London 1977).
57 Winchester, J.F.: Haemostatic changes induced by adsorbent haemoperfusion; in Kenedi, Cortney, Gaylor, Gilchrist, Artificial organs, p. 280 (Macmillan Press, London 1977).
58 Winchester, J.F.; MacKay, J.M.; Forbes, C.D.; Courtney, J.M.; Gilchrist, T.; Prentice, C.R.M.: Hemostatic changes induced in vitro by hemoperfusion over activated charcoal. Artif. Organs *2:* 293 (1978).
59 Winchester, J.F.; Ratcliffe, J.D.; Carlyle, E.; Kennedy, A.C.: Solute amino acid, and hormone changes with coated charcoal hemoperfusion in uremia. Kidney int. *14:* 74 (1978).
60 Yatzidis, H.: A convenient haemoperfusion micro-apparatus over charcoal for the treatment of endogenous and exogenous intoxications. Its use as effective artificial kidney. Proc. Eur. Dialysis Transplant. Ass. *1:* 83 (1964).

T. Gilchrist, PhD, Bioengineering Unit, University of Strathclyde, Glasgow (Scotland)

Contr. Nephrol., vol. 29, pp. 53–64 (Karger, Basel 1982)

Sorbent Membrane Dialysis in Uremia[1]

D.H. Randerson[a], H.J. Gurland[a], B. Schmidt[a], P.C. Farrell[e], P.W.E. Hone[e], C. Stokoe[e], A. Zuber[e], A. Blogg[e], A. Fateh-Moghadam[b], I. Marschner[c], W. Köpcke[d]

[a] Medizinische Klinik I, Klinikum Grosshadern;
[b] Institut für Klinische Chemie, Klinikum Grosshadern;
[c] Medizinische Klinik Innenstadt;
[d] Institut für Medizinische Informationsverarbeitung, Statistik und Biomathematik, Klinikum Grosshadern, Universität München, FRG;
[e] Centre for Biomedical Engineering, University of New South Wales, Sydney, Australia

Introduction

The hypothesis that uremic symptoms in dialysis patients may result from the retention of substances in the middle molecular weight range (300–2,000 Daltons) [1] has resulted in considerable change to conventional hemodialysis (HD) regimens over the past 10 years. Developments include more porous membranes and hemofiltration both enabling improved middle molecule clearance. *Chang* et al. [2] suggested activated charcoal as a possible adsorbent for 'middle molecules', and in 1975 [3] reported on the substitution of one of three weekly HD sessions with charcoal hemoperfusion – hemodialysis on a long-term basis. The simultaneous application of hemoperfusion and hemodialysis was also reported by *Winchester* et al. [20] in 1975 and in the following year by *Odaka* et al. [16]. Such procedures although effective in improving creatinine and middle molecule removal were, however, cumbersome and costly.

Sorbent membranes, for combined dialytic and adsorptive removal of solute, were developed by Enka AG (Wuppertal, FRG) in 1976 and have since been incorporated into prototype dialyzer configuration (Medical Incorporated, Minnesota, and Gambro Dialysatoren GmbH, FRG). The flat sheet sorbent membrane consists of a Cuprophan® layer (9 μm) (forming the blood interface) backed by a second layer (50 μm) of cellulose impregnated with activated charcoal, 18 g of charcoal per m^2 membrane surface area.

[1] Supported by grants from Enka AG, Wuppertal, FRG.

In vitro evaluations [10, 11] have shown that urea clearance per unit membrane surface area is not compromised by the additional cellulose layer. Initial clearances of creatinine and phenobarbital were found to be significantly enhanced (20–25% in the case of creatinine, and 70–110% for phenobarbital) by the charcoal adsorption. Clearances in the middle molecule range (digoxin, vitamin B_{12} and inulin) were also significantly improved. However, as the adsorption capacity of charcoal is limited, clearances of creatinine and phenobarbital decreased progressively during the first hours of in vitro operation [11, 18], which may restrict long-term application to renal replacement therapy.

Long-term crossover studies (comparing HD and sorbent membrane dialysis; SMD) are necessary to assess the efficacy of SMD for the treatment of patients with end-stage renal disease. This paper reports on 2 independently conducted trials.

Materials and Methods

Munich Study

In vitro dialyzer clearances were measured using a synthetic blood of standard dialysate (282 mosm/l) with the relevant radiolabelled test substances added. Experiments were conducted at 37 °C with 8 liters of 'blood' recirculated at 200 ml/min, and dialyzed against single pass standard dialysate at 500 ml/min. Clearances were obtained for each solute individually over a 4-hour 'dialysis'. Carrier solute concentrations were: urea 16.7 m*M*/l, creatinine 0.88 m*M*/l, phenobarbital 0.43 m*M*/l, vitamin B_{12} 0.092 μ*M*/l, and inulin 0.12 m*M*/l.

14 patients who had been stable on dialysis for at least 6 months were selected for a long-term crossover study comparing sorbent (Sorbiclear, Medical Incorporated, Minnesota, A = 1.28 m^2) and conventional Cuprophan dialysis (Gambro Lundia Optima, Gambro, Sweden, A = 1.0 m^2). The patients were randomly divided into 2 groups of 7 patients following an A-B-A or a B-A-B program, where 'A' was conventional HD and 'B' SMD. Each period lasted for 3 months. Treatment times for all patients were 4 h 3 times per week on both modalities.

Patient selection criteria included: (i) residual clearance <3.0 ml/min; (ii) urinary output <500 ml/day; (iii) interdialytic weight gain <2.5 kg; (iv) body weight deviation from ideal <20%; (v) serum potassium <6.5 m*M*/l; (vi) serum phosphate <3.0m*M*/l; (vii) no arterial hypertension; (viii) no bilateral nephrectomy; (ix) no secondary disease; (x) age between 25 and 65 years; (xi) in-center dialysis.

39 biochemical and clinical parameters were investigated either weekly, monthly, or 3-monthly (i.e. at the end of each study period). The majority of serum samples and especially those taken once every 3 months were determined in a single preparation in order to keep analytical errors to a minimum. Predialysis, midweek serum samples were used for all analyses.

The results were assessed by analysis of variance according to the method described by *Finney* [6]. A computer program (CROSS) written by the National Institute for Biological Standards and Control [8] was used to process data. The program is written for a crossover 2 × 2 format (ie. patient group I A-B, group II B-A), and in order to process the data of the SMD/HD study it was necessary to perform two analyses – treatment periods I and II (group

I A-B, group II B-A) and periods II and III (group I B-A, group II A-B). Significance was required in both analyses, however no discrepancies were observed. For each parameter used in the computation, patient means were used where more than one set of data had been obtained during the study period.

Sydney Study

A 13-month study was designed to assess the efficacy of hemofiltration and SMD (Sorbiclear) in comparison with conventional dialysis (MTS C1.0 Hemoflow, Fresenius, FRG, A = 1.0 m^2). Using well-established [13, 14] procedures they assessed in vitro performance of the Sorbiclear and MTS C1.0 dialyzers. Clearances were measured for a spectrum of radiolabelled solutes using single pass procedures, at 37 ± 0.1 °C with 0.15 *M* saline flowing countercurrently in both blood and dialysate compartments at flow rates of 200 and 500 ml/min, respectively, and transmembrane pressure zero. Carrier solute concentrations were: urea 0.83 m*M*/l, creatinine 0.44 m*M*/l, sucrose 0.15 m*M*/l and vitamin B_{12} 0.0074 m*M*/l. Blood and dialysate side clearances were measured within 5 min of adding tagged solute.

To assess the influence of membrane saturation on the clearance of a highly charcoal-adsorbed solute, new Sorbiclear dialyzers were continously perfused at 200 ml/min with saline containing 1.0 m*M*/l of creatinine carrier and labelled with 3 μCi/l of ^{14}C-creatinine. Dialysate flow was controlled to 500 ml/min and transmembrane pressure was adjusted to 60 mm Hg to ensure expansion of all blood channels. In vitro blood-side and dialysate-side clearances were measured at regular intervals.

8 patients were selected for the crossover study complying with the following criteria: all patients (i) were stabilized on HD for at least 3 months prior to the study; (ii) were clinically well with no secondary diseases; (iii) had blood access capable of achieving 200 ml/min on a routine basis, and (iv) had residual renal function less than 2.0 ml/min.

Patients were stabilized with at least 4 weeks control dialysis, during which period they were modelled for heparin requirements [5] (which were subsequently reviewed monthly) and dialysis times (TD) reduced to give midweek predialysis serum urea levels of approximately 33 m*M*/l in each patient.

4 patients were dialyzed on an A-B-A-C-A protocol and 4 on an A-C-A-B-A protocol. Regimen 'A' was an 8-week control period of 3 × TD h/week conventional dialysis. 'B' was SMD, 3 × TD h/week for 14 weeks, and 'C' 3 × TD h/week for 14 weeks of hemodiafiltration (Nipro F-1 Hemofilter, Nisho Corp., Tokyo). During the entire study blood and dialysate flows were maintained as close as possible to 200 and 500 ml/min, respectively.

Routine biochemical and hematological samples were collected immediately prior to the midweek dialysis on a monthly basis. Net urea and creatinine generation rates were determined using a single-pool, variable-volume model [4], requiring pre-, post- and pre-data from two consecutive dialyses. Assuming patients to be in nitrogen balance, the protein catabolic rate (PCR) was calculated from urea generation using a correlation derived by *Gotch* et al. [9]. Generation rates and PCRs were measured every 4th week. At least once during each treatment regimen a dietary survey was conducted to coincide with measurement of urea generation rates. Complete records of dietary intake during a 1-week period were kept by each patient and an interview with a trained renal dietician was conducted to verify whether the record was representative of the period as a whole and to specify details of food intake.

In vivo dialyzer clearances were measured every 4th week using previously described methods [19].

For this report data from the two crossover groups were combined as A-B-A, and the two treatments compared by the paired Student's t test.

Table I. In vitro clearance[1] data of dialyzers used in the Munich study.

Solute	Dialyzer	Time, min				
		5	15	30	60	240
Urea	Sorbiclear	137 ± 9	138 ± 8	137 ± 9	136 ± 11	140 ± 6
	Optima	134 ± 9	132 ± 6	135 ± 7	132 ± 5	128 ± 9
Creatinine	Sorbiclear	135 ± 6	119 ± 2	105 ± 5	100 ± 8	82 ± 8
	Optima	98 ± 2	94 ± 9	104 ± 5	106 ± 5	100 ± 10
Pheno-	Sorbiclear	141 ± 15	127 ± 12	114 ± 8	87 ± 6	62 ± 7
barbital	Optima	73 ± 1	75 ± 2	77 ± 3	80 ± 2	74 ± 3
Vitamin	Sorbiclear	51 ± 3	51 ± 0.3	51 ± 4	48 ± 7	43 ± 6
B_{12}	Optima	28 ± 4	27 ± 1	21 ± 8	26 ± 5	23 ± 4
Inulin	Sorbiclear	16 ± 4	19 ± 5	16 ± 6	14 ± 5	9 ± 2
	Optima	6 ± 2	5 ± 5	8 ± 3	9 ± 1	4 ± 1

[1] ml/min, mean ± SD (Sorbiclear, n = 4; Gambro Optima, n = 2), Q_B = 200 ml/min, Q_D = 500 ml/min, UFR = 0.

Table II. In vitro performance of dialyzers used in the Sydney study

Dialyzer	Clearance, ml/min[1]				Ultrafiltration (ml/h)
	urea	creatinine	sucrose	vitamin B_{12}	at 100 mm/Hg TMP
Sorbiclear (n = 3)	126 ± 4	155 ± 4	102 ± 3	57 ± 4	350 ± 15
MTS C1.0 Hemoflow (n = 7)	151 ± 16	124 ± 15	76 ± 12	31 ± 5	320 ± 11

[1] Q_B = 200 ml/min, Q_D = 500 ml/min, UFR = 0.

Results and Discussion

In vitro Studies

Gurland et al. [10, 11] have published in vitro comparisons of sorbent membrane dialyzers with standard hemodialyzers. The data for the Gambro Lundia Optima and the Sorbiclear are reproduced in table I. The results show that urea clearances for the two devices are similar even though the Sorbiclear has 30% greater surface area suggesting greater transport resistance due to the additional

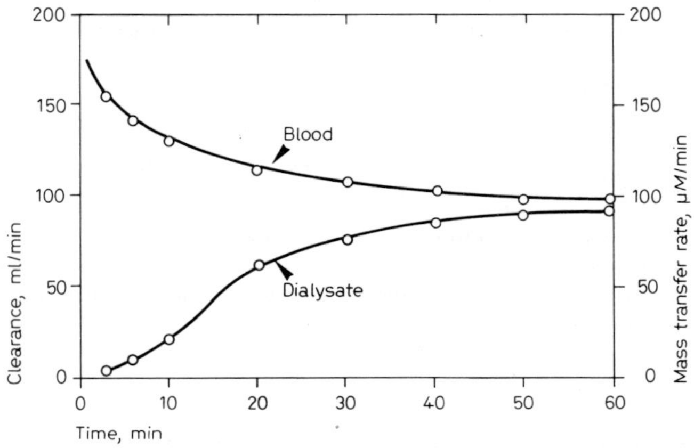

Fig. 1. In vitro clearance and mass transfer rates for the Sorbiclear dialyzer during its 1st h of use.

cellulose layer. Clearances of creatinine and phenobarbital were initially significantly higher with SMD, but declined progressively due to saturation of the charcoal. At 1 h for creatinine, and 3 for phenobarbital, the adsorption sites were apparently saturated and only standard dialysis occurred.

For the two substances in the middle molecular weight range, vitamin B_{12} and inulin, significantly higher clearances with sorbent membrane devices were found. Clearances of both substances declined with time although considerable charcoal adsorption was still apparent after 4 h.

Results of the Sydney in vitro dialyzer evaluations are presented in table II. Although Sorbiclear urea clearance was relatively poor due to a low charcoal affinity for urea, its ability to clear species highly adsorbed to charcoal (creatinine and vitamin B_{12}) was impressive, in agreement with the Munich data.

Mean creatinine clearances and mass tranfer rates as functions of time are shown in figure 1. The differences between rate of mass transfer from blood-side and the rate of transfer into dialysate at any time corresponds to the rate of adsorption on the sorbent membrane. The area between the two rate curves on figure 1 is equivalent to the amount of solute adsorbed by the membrane. With a constant 'blood' creatinine concentration the rate of adsorption rapidly decreases and the sorbent membrane is close to saturation after as little as 1 h of dialysis. At this point the creatinine clearances are 96 ± 3 ml/min and a total of

Table III. In vivo[1] dialyzer clearances obtained during the Sydney study (mean ± SD)

Dialyzer	Clearance, ml/min		UFR, ml/min	Q_B, ml/min	Q_D, ml/min
	urea	creatinine			
Sorbiclear (n = 48)	113 ± 12	91 ± 7	9.2 ± 3.0	201 ± 14	498 ± 16
MTS C1.0 (n = 86)	166 ± 9	130 ± 12	9.1 ± 3.1	199 ± 9	504 ± 25

[1] Determined 1 h after commencing and 1 h prior to termination of dialysis

5.6 ± 0.8 m*M* of creatinine has been adsorbed by the 23 g of activated charcoal contained within the Sorbiclear. Approximately 20 m*M* of creatinine is normally removed from patients on thrice weekly dialysis and if dialyzer clearances are to be effectively enhanced, a considerably higher charcoal content is required.

Although the blood creatinine level gradually falls during actual dialysis there are many charcoal-adsorbed species, such as amino acids, which cross the dialyzer membrane and are likely to compete with creatinine uptake. This process would be expected to accelerate the fall in creatinine clearance during the first hour. Clearly, for the major portion of dialysis the charcoal actually contributes to the membrane's mass transfer resistance rather than solute removal. However, there may be a trade-off if a much thinner, more permeable membrane could be used with a charcoal support.

In vivo Dialyzer Clearances

The Sydney study involved measuring in vivo dialyzer clearances of urea and creatinine using methods described by *Skalsky* et al. [19]. These were performed 1 h after commencing and 1 h prior to termination of dialysis at monthly intervals. Clearances for each dialyzer are combined as means ± standard deviations in table III. Blood and dialysate flow rates have been set as close as possible to 200 and 500 ml/min, while ultrafiltration rates were adjusted to suit patient requirements. Clearances have not been corrected for small deviations in flow rate and are enhanced by the ultrafiltration rate.

In vivo Sorbiclear clearances of urea and creatinine are slightly lower than the values expected for 9.2 ml/min of ultrafiltration after 1 hours use. This, together with a further decline in performance after 2.5 hours suggests that either membrane stretching or thrombus formation is occuring within the Sorbiclear during use. Although both factors may be responsible for a progressive decline in urea and creatinine clearances, membrane stretching is suspected here as it is known to occur in most dialyzers of parallel plate construction. It is a fault in Sorbiclear design rather than in sorbent membrane manufacture.

The MTS C1.0 in vivo clearances of both urea and creatinine (table III) agree closely with the in vitro values obtained in table II when allowance is made for the UFR.

In vivo UFRs of 325 and 320 ml/h at 100 m Hg TMP were routinely estimated for Sorbiclear and MTS C1.0 dialyzers, respectively. Both values are in good agreement with respective in vitro values of 350 and 320 ml/h.

Results of Crossover Studies

Results of the Munich crossover study are presented in table IV. Significant differences were observed in serum levels of urea (30.2 ± 4.0 m*M*/l SMD cf. 26.3 ± 3.0 m*M*/l HD), creatinine (1.17 ± 0.12 m*M*/l SMD cf. 1.02 ± 0.12 m*M*/l HD), inorganic phosphate (1.99 ± 0.31 m*M*/l SMD cf. 1.68 ± 0.22 m*M*/l HD), cholesterol (5.0 ± 1.0 m*M*/l SMD cf. 5.4 ± 1.1 m*M*/l HD), and middle molecule peak 'b' (1,350 ± 550 cm^2 peak area/ml SMD cf. 1,100 ± 500 cm^2/ml HD). No other parameters displayed significant variance between dialysis regimens.

Results of the Sydney study are presented in table V. Average dialysis times for the Sydney group (see 'Materials and Methods') were 3.4 ± 0.4 h/treatment (range 2.0–4.0 h) adjusted to give a mean midweek predialysis HD urea level of approximately 33 m*M*/l. Significant differences between treatments were observed for creatinine (1.31 ± 0.21 m*M*/l SMD cf. 1.19 ± 2.5 m*M*/l HD), serum alkaline phosphatase (86 ± 30 IU/l SMD cf. 100 ± 54 IU/l HD), and magnesium (1.22 ± 0.14 m*M*/l SMD cf. 1.14 ± 0.13 m*M*/l HD).

The findings of the two independently conducted crossover studies suggest no major advantages of SMD over conventional HD with regard to biochemical parameters and medical investigations. There is no improvement in creatinine levels and, if anything, they tended to be worse on SMD. Serum urea and phosphate levels were also found to be elevated on SMD, probably a consequence of reduced clearance of these moieties. Phosphate binder intakes were held constant during all study periods in both studies. SMD may also lead to a marginal increase in magnesium levels when compared to conventional dialysis. The reason for this is obscure and the clinical significance of elevated serum magnesium is unknown. Reduced cholesterol levels observed in the Munich study may be an advantage of SMD. The reason for the reduced alkaline phosphatase level in the Sydney study is unknown.

One of the purported advantages of SMD is higher middle molecule removal; however, the data obtained in the Munich study suggest that if anything middle molecule levels are probably worse. This may result from competitive binding on the charcoal. Peak 'b' has been found to be elevated in patients with neuropathy [7]; however, nerve conduction velocities showed no significant differences. In contrast to the Munich results, *Lindsay* et al. [15] in a 6-month crossover study

Table IV. Results of the Munich crossover study (mean ± SD, n = 21)

	SMD	HD
Parameters determined once a week		
Urea, m*M*/l	30.2 ± 4.0*	26.3 ± 3.0
Creatinine, m*M*/l	1.17 ± 0.12*	1.02 ± 0.12
Potassium, m*M*/l	5.6 ± 0.2	5.5 ± 0.2
Hemoglobin, g/dl	8.2 ± 1.0	8.3 ± 0.9
Hematocrit, %	26.8 ± 2.8	26.1 ± 2.4
Leukocytes, $\times 10^9$/l	6.7 ± 1.5	6.4 ± 1.3
Thrombocytes, $\times 10^9$/l	170 ± 31	163 ± 21
Weight, kg (post-dx)	64.8 ± 6.0	63.0 ± 6.7
Parameters determined once a month		
Calcium, m*M*/l	2.2 ± 0.9	2.2 ± 0.8
Phosphate, m*M*/l	1.99 ± 0.31*	1.68 ± 0.22
Alkaline phospatase IU/l	194 ± 46	174 ± 40
Cholesterol, m*M*/l	5.0 ± 1.0*	5.4 ± 1.1
Triglyceride, m*M*/l	2.2 ± 0.7	2.2 ± 0.7
Iron, μM/l	20 ± 9	14 ± 2
pH	7.35 ± 0.20	7.37 ± 0.31
pO_2, mm Hg	95 ± 7	94 ± 10
pCO_2, mm Hg	31 ± 7	31 ± 14
Bicarbonate, m*M*/l	17 ± 8	18 ± 9
Base excess, m*M*/l	−7.4 ± 0.4	−6.8 ± 1.1
Nerve conduction velocity, m/s		
Peroneal	39 ± 4	40 ± 3
Ulnar	48 ± 3	48 ± 4

*Significance, $p < 0.05$.

found a greater removal of plasma middle molecules with sorbent membrane dialysis. *Oulès* et al. [17] measured middle molecule uptake during 3-hour charcoal hemoperfusions of uremic patients using a Gambro hemoperfusion column (Adsorba 300 C), containing 300 g of cellulose-encapsulated activated charcoal. Initially high extraction levels gradually decreased during the perfusion and two middle molecule fractions (peaks 7a and 7b) showed evidence of release from the column during the final hour of perfusion. The results suggest competitive adsorption of substance(s) in serum is displacing these middle molecule fractions. Middle molecule levels were also measured in the Sydney study. Results are not available as yet.

During the Sydney study both caloric and protein intakes, as assessed by the renal dietician, remained fairly constant, and creatinine generation, a marker for muscle mass, and postdialysis body weight remained stable. However, there may

Table IV. (continued)

	SMD	HD
Parameters determined 3 monthly		
Total protein, g/l	71 ± 3	71 ± 3
Pre-albumin. g/l	3 ± 2.1	2 ± 1.3
Electrophoresis		
albumin, %	61.8 ± 3.6	60.8 ± 3.5
α_1, %	3.3 ± 7.5	3.1 ± 5.6
α_2, %	7.4 ± 1.0	7.7 ± 0.9
β, %	8.1 ± 0.9	8.3 ± 0.9
γ, %	18.7 ± 3.1	18.1 ± 2.9
IgA, g/l	2.2 ± 0.7	2.0 ± 0.9
IgG, g/l	10.1 ± 1.8	10.0 ± 1.7
IgM, g/l	0.8 ± 0.3	0.9 ± 0.3
PTH, ng/ml	4.6 ± 1.3	4.0 ± 1.3
Middle molecule peak 'b', cm^2/ml[1]	1,350 ± 550*	1,100 ± 500
Transferrin, g/l	2.5 ± 0.3	2.5 ± 0.3
Complement C_3, g/l	0.74 ± 0.12	0.70 ± 0.06
SGPT, IU/l	10.8 ± 2.6	11.5 ± 3.6
SGOT, IU/l	11.9 ± 2.7	9.9 ± 1.9
Retinol binding protein, mg/l	24.7 ± 2.7	25.8 ± 3.4
Radiographic bone densitometry[2]	77 ± 11	76 ± 12

* Significance, $p < 0.05$.

[1] Determined by gel chromatography (Sephadex G15) following the method of *Funck-Brentano* et al. [7].

[2] Determined by Radiological Research Laboratory, Greene Memorial Hospital Inc., Ohio.

have been a slight decrease in urea generation and computed PCR. The suppression is possibly due to the elevated serum urea level.

Neither hemoglobin levels nor packed cell volumes were affected by SMD. Platelet and leukocyte counts were also stable. Blood pressures were well controlled.

Conclusions

Sorbent membrane dialysis was found to be less effective than conventional HD in controlling metabolite levels in uremia and appears to offer no advantages over HD. Creatinine levels and middle molecule levels do not decrease as anticipated due to charcoal saturation coupled with low dialytic clearance of the Sor-

Table V. Results of the crossover study

	SMD (n = 16)	HD (n = 8)
Sodium, m*M*/l	140 ± 2	139 ± 2
Potassium, m*M*/l	4.9 ± 0.4	4.8 ± 0.6
Chloride, m*M*/l	97 ± 3	98 ± 3
Bicarbonate, m*M*/l	24 ± 2	24 ± 3
Phosphate, m*M*/l	1.84 ± 0.36	1.66 ± 0.51
Calcium, m*M*/l	2.44 ± 0.19	2.44 ± 0.21
Magnesium, m*M*/l	1.22 ± 0.14*	1.14 ± 0.13
Alkaline phosphatase IU/l	86 ± 30*	100 ± 54
Albumin, g/l	40 ± 2	41 ± 2
Total protein, g/l	70 ± 3	70 ± 4
Urea, m*M*/l	31.9 ± 6.7	27.5 ± 6.7
Creatinine, m*M*/l	1.31 ± 0.21*	1.19 ± 0.25
Urate, mM/l	0.52 ± 0.05	0.50 ± 0.05
Bilirubin, μM/l	7 ± 1	6 ± 2
Hemoglobin, g/l	7.5 ± 1.3	7.5 ± 1.1
Hematocrit, %	22.9 ± 3.5	23.3 ± 3.1
Leukocytes, $\times 10^9$/l	5.1 ± 1.3	4.9 ± 1.3
Weight, kg (post-dx)	56.8 ± 14.7	56.8 ± 14.1
Diastolic BP, mm Hg		
Pre-dx	80 ± 14	83 ± 15
Post-dx	72 ± 16	73 ± 16
Dietary protein intake, g/day[1]	54.9 ± 7.7	54.7 ± 9.2
Dietary caloric intake, kcal/day[1]	1580 ± 350	1620 ± 330
Urea generation rate, μM/min	140 ± 30	170 ± 40
Protein catabolic rate, g/day[2]	51 ± 10	60 ± 13
Creatinine generation rate, μm/day	6.3 ± 2.3	6.2 ± 1.8

* Significance, $p < 0.05$.
[1] Determined by 1 week dietary survey.
[2] Determined from urea generation rate using correlation derived by *Gotch* et al. [9].

biclear device. The results suggest that the 23 g of activated charcoal in the existing device are insufficient to compensate for the reduced dialytic removal and that an increased carbon content would be necessary to effect any advantages over HD.

The use of sorbent membrane dialyzers in the treatment of end-stage renal disease must be viewed in relation to the relative cost compared to HD. However, it may find application in liver support, exogenous intoxications, psoriasis, etc. as discussed by *Gurland* [12].

Summary

The inclusion of activated charcoal within hemodialysis membranes offers potentially improved plasma clearance of creatinine and middle molecules. However, the carbon becomes saturated with continued use and beyond 1 h removal of solutes is by dialysis alone. Two independently conducted crossover studies, to assess the efficacy of sorbent membrane dialysis (SMD) in the treatment of uremia, found predialysis urea levels increased by approximately 15%, creatinine by 10–15%, and inorganic phosphate levels by 10–18% on SMD compared to conventional hemodialysis. One study also observed 'middle molecule' (peak 'b') levels elevated. No differences were observable in the clinical status of patients. The results suggest that the charcoal content of the SMD device is too small to effect any advantages over conventional dialysis.

References

1 Babb, A.L.; Farrell, P.C.; Uvelli, D.A.; Scribner, B.H.: Hemodialyzer evaluation by examination of solute molecular spectra. Trans. Am. Soc. artif. internal Organs *18:* 98–105 (1972).

2 Chang, T.M.S.; Migchelson, M.; Coffey, J.F.; Stark, A.: Serum middle molecule levels in uremia during long-term intermittent hemoperfusion with the ACAC coated charcoal microcapsule artificial kidney. Trans. Am. Soc. artif. internal Organs *20:* 364–372 (1974).

3 Chang, T.M.S.; Chirito, E.; Barre, P.; Cole, C.; Hewish, M.: Clinical performance characteristics of a new combined system for simultaneous hemoperfusion-hemodialysis-ultrafiltration in series. Trans. Am. Soc. artif. internal Organs *21:* 502–508 (1975).

4 Farrell, P.C.; Gotch, F.A.: Dialysis therapy guided by kinetic modelling: Applications of a variable-volume single pool model of urea kinetics. Proc. Australasian Conf. Heat Mass Transf. *2:* 29–34 (1977).

5 Farrell, P.C.; Ward, R.A.; Schindhelm, K.; Gotch, F.A.: Precise anticoagulation for routine hemodialysis. J. Lab. clin. Med. *92:* 164–169 (1978).

6 Finney, D.J.: Statistical method in biologic assay, chap. 10, pp. 265–299 (Griffin, London 1964).

7 Funck-Brentano, J.L.; Man, N.K.; Sausse, A.; Zingraff, J.; Boudet, J.; Becker, A.; Cueille, G.F.: Characterisation of a 1100–1300 MW uremic neurotoxin. Trans. Am. Soc. artif. internal Organs *22:* 163–167 (1976).

8 Gaines-Das, R.E.; Hughes, M.R.: A computer program for the analysis of crossover designs. Comp. Prog. Biomed. *10:* 105–113 (1979).

9 Gotch, F.A.; Sargent, J.A.; Keen, M.L.; Lam, M.; Prowitt, M.; Grady, M.: Solute kinetics of intermittent dialysis therapy. Proc. Ann. Contractors' Conf. AK-NIAMDD *9:* 98–101 (1976).

10 Gurland, H.J.; Fernandez, J.C.; Samtleben, W.; Castro, L.A.: Sorbent membranes used in a conventional dialyzer format. Artif. Organs *2:* 372–374 (1978).

11 Gurland, H.J.; Castro, L.A.; Samtleben, W.; Fernandez, J.C.: Combination of hemodialysis and hemoperfusion in a single unit for treatment of uremia. Clin. Nephrol. *11:* 167–172 (1979).

12 Gurland, H.J.: Combination of hemodialysis and hemoperfusion used in conventional dialyzer format in the treatment of uremia. Proc. Ann. Contractors' Conf. AK-NIAMDD, *12:* 279–287 (1979).

13 Hone, P.W.E.; Ward, R.A.; Mahony, J.F.; Farrell, P.C.: Hemodialyzer performance. An assessment of currently available units. J. Dial. *1:* 285–290 (1977).
14 Hone, P.W.E.; Randerson, D.H.; Farrell, P.C.: Performance characteristics of disposable dialyzers. Dial. Transpl. *8:* 689–691 (1979).
15 Lindsay, R.M.; Cvejich, L.; Clark, F.; Linton, A.C.: The evaluation of combined hemodialysis-hemoperfusion system. Abstr. Eur. Dial. Transpl. Ass. XVIth Congress, 1979, p. 54.
16 Odaka, M.; Tabata, Y.; Kobayashi, H.; Nomura, Y.; Soma, M.; Hirasawa, H.; Sato, H.; Suenaga, E.; Nabeta, K.: Three hour maintenance dialysis combining direct hemoperfusion and hemodialysis. Proc. Eur. Dial. Transpl. Ass. *13:* 257–261 (1976).
17 Oulès, R.; Asaba, H.; Neuhäuser, M.; Yahiel, V.; Gunnarsson, B.; Bergström, J.; Fürst, P.: The removal of uremic small and middle molecules and free amino acids by carbon hemoperfusion. Trans. Am. Soc. artif. internal Organs *23:* 588–589 (1977).
18 Özdural, A.R.; Piskin, E.: Sorbent membranes: Determination of sorbent capacity and true membrane permeability. Artif. Organs *4:* 322–325 (1980).
19 Skalsky, M.; Schindhelm, K.; Farrell, P.C.: Accurate determinations of in vivo dialyzer clearances. Dial. Transpl. *7:* 1217–1221 (1978).
20 Winchester, J.F.; Apiliga, M.T.; Mackay, J.M.; Kennedy, A.C.: Haemodialysis with charcoal haemoperfusion. Proc. Eur. Dial. Transpl. Ass. *12:* 526–531 (1975).

Prof. Dr. med. H.J. Gurland, Medizinische Klinik I, Nephrology Division
Klinikum Grosshadern, University of Munich, P.O. Box 701 260,
D–8000 Munich 70 (FRG)

Contr. Nephrol., vol. 29, pp. 65–75 (Karger, Basel 1982)

Use of Uncoated Activated Carbon Hemoperfusion in Acute Poisoning: In vitro Studies

Vincenzo Tessore[a], *M.P. Luboz*[a], *Ennio Denti*[b]

[a] Sorin Biomedica SpA, and
[b] National Research Council, Special Program on Biomedical Technology, Subproject Farm-3, Saluggia, Italy

Introduction

The removal of toxin from the blood stream could be done using extracorporeal detoxification techniques as, for example, hemodialysis, hemofiltration, ultrafiltration and hemoperfusion. The simplest approach to the problem is the use of hemoperfusion.

The first clinical experiments of blood detoxification by extracorporeal circulation through columns of activated carbon were conducted in 1964 by *Yatzidis* [1]. He found that activated carbon could effectively remove endogenous and exogenous toxins. Subsequent experiments conducted by several investigators showed the efficacy of this procedure but also pointed out the occurrence of undesired side effects. Later work by *Dunea and Kolff* [2] reported that platelets were reduced by 50%, and *Hagstam* et al. [3, 4] found carbon particles in the lungs, liver and kidneys in animal perfusion studies. Figure 1 clearly shows the presence in pulmonary tissue of a rabbit of a carbon particle subsequent to an experimental hemoperfusion. In order to face this problem, several investigators [5–11] tried to minimize the particle release by coating the sorbent with different polymeric membranes. Generally speaking the effect of those membranes was a reduction in the carbon particles generation, a reduction in absorption rate of the sorbent, and in some cases, an improvement on blood compatibility of the sorbent. Figure 2 shows the effect of regenerated cellulose coating on the absorption behavior of Columbia LCK-activated carbon.

Hill et al. [12] devised a completely different approach in order to solve the problem of microparticles release immobilizing the charcoal granules on a special adhesive tape coiled and inserted in a cylindrical container. This device, called 'Hemodetoxifier' (Becton & Dickinson), clearly showed the possibility to avoid microparticles generation reducing the attrition between sorbent particles.

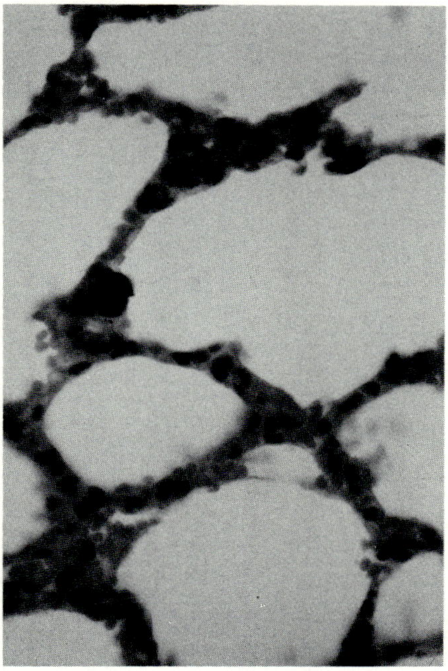

Fig. 1. Carbon microparticles in lung tissue.

Carbon Selection

Another obvious approach to reduce particles generation without coating could be to use activated carbons characterized by a high surface hardness. The criteria for activated carbon selection were already described elsewhere [13]. Utilizing material characterized by low attrition resistance and organizing it in an appropriate container it could be possible to manufacture a hemoperfusion column with very low microparticles generation and high absorption rate.

Materials and Methods

Column preparation

The activated carbon utilized in the hemoperfusion columns is the spherical type Bac-Mu manufactured by Taiyo Kaken Co. Ltd. (fig. 3). The column (250 mm length, 36 mm diameter) was manufactured utilizing blow moulded polypropylene. The caps and internal retention mesh were made of medical grade polypropylene. In order to avoid movement and consequently attrition between the carbon particles, 2 small cylindrical filters of polyure-

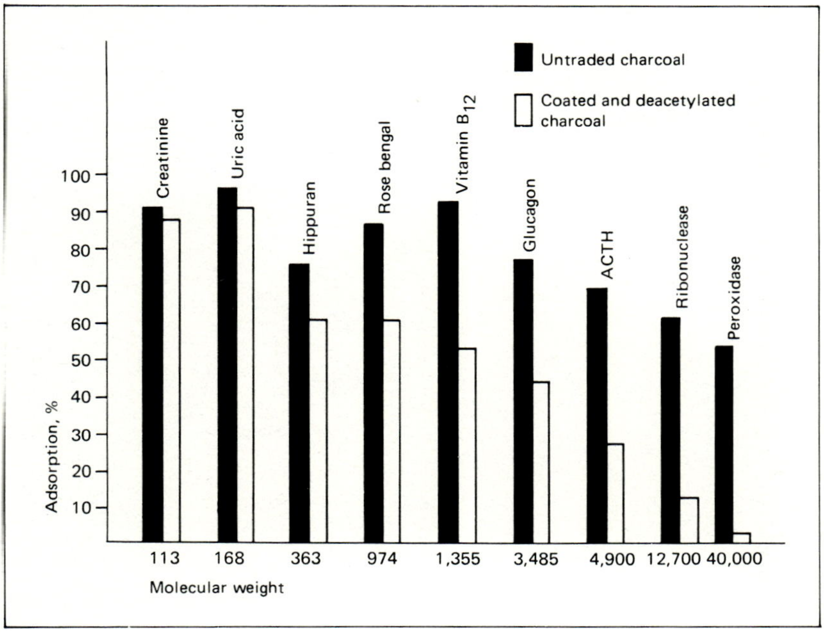

Fig. 2. Test molecules adsorption of coated and uncoated Columbia LCK-activated carbon.

thane foam, open porosity, were inserted, slightly compressed at the top and bottom of the columns. The activated carbon was washed carefully utilizing deionized and sterile water in a fluidized bed obtained circulating the water at the appropriate speed into a vertical cylindrical Plexiglas container. After this washing procedure, the column was filled pouring the carbon/water slurry into the column and utilizing the same maneuvers done for the preparation of chromatographic columns. Finally the top polyurethane foam filter and the propylene mesh is put in place and the propylene cap inserted.

Following this step the column was submitted to a washing procedure with 0.9% NaCl solution utilizing a peristaltic pump recirculating for 1 h at mean flow rate of 200 ml/min. In order to favor the elimination of any eventual microparticle trapped into the columns, the peristaltic pump works with the tubing completely occluded while the suction tube is fitted with a 14-gauge needle for obtaining a pulsatile flow. After this preparation, the column is submitted to sterilization by exposure to gamma radiation with a dosage of 2.5 Mrad.

Clearance Determination

The clearance of the columns was assessed by perfusing an aqueous solution of creatinine, inulin, phenobarbital, uric acid, glucose, urea, vitamin B_{12}, salicyclic acid, through 2 columns in series at a flow rate of 200 ± 10 ml/min.

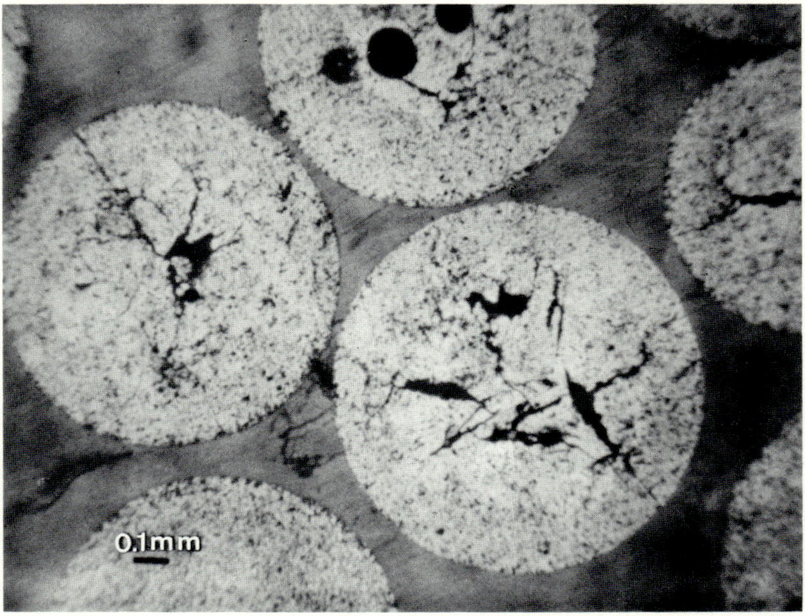

Fig. 3. Cross section of Bac-Mu-activated carbon. × 52.5.

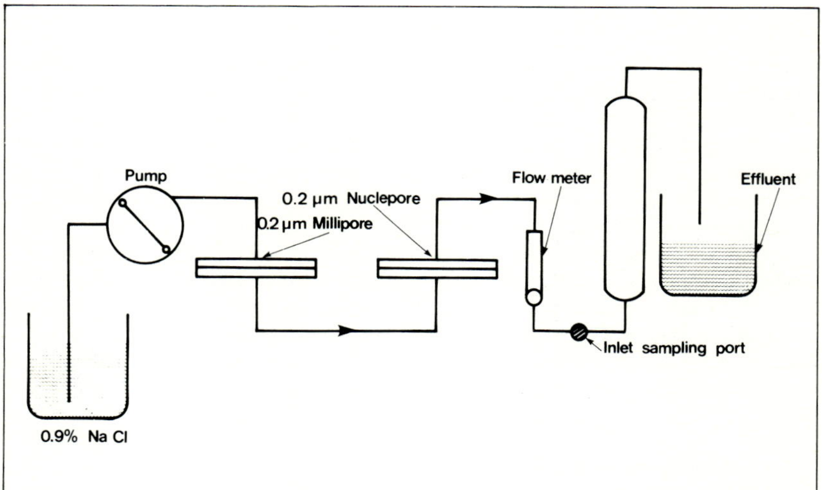

Fig. 4. Experimental set-up for microparticles determination.

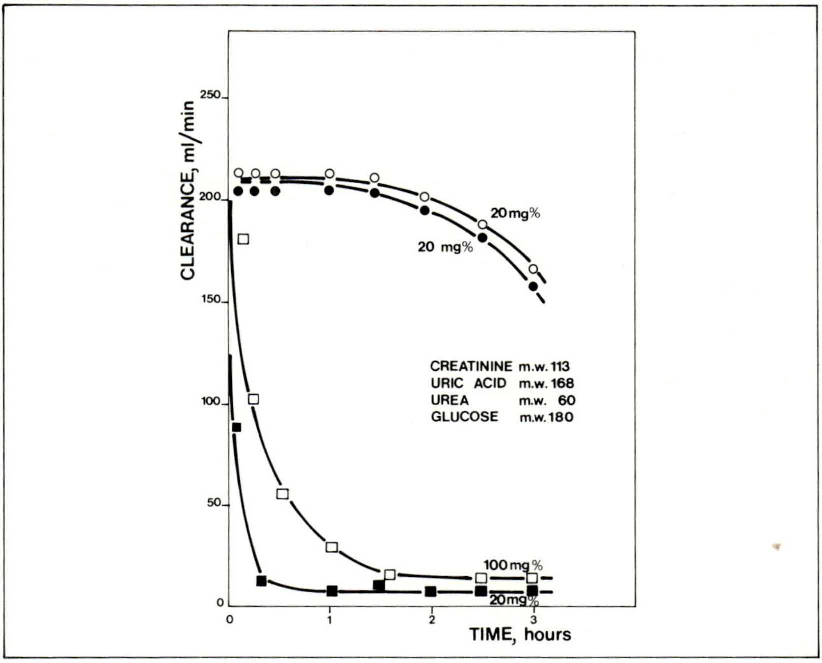

Fig. 5. Clearances vs. time of two detoxyl 2 columns in series for some test molecules.

Microparticle Generation

The microparticle determination was done utilizing a Coulter counter model D (Industrial) manufactured by Coulter Electronic Ltd., England. Figure 4 shows the experimental set-up utilized for the microparticle determination. In order to avoid as much as possible the generation of microparticles from the polyvinyl chloride segment of the peristaltic pump system, the pump is followed by 0.2-μm Millipore filter and subsequently 0.2-μm Nuclepore filter. Samples of saline were taken at the column inlet and from 1 liter effluent after washing the column with 1 liter saline. The inlet and effluent samples were analyzed by a Coulter counter.

Analytical Procedures

The following analytical methods were used:

(1) C. Erba autoanalyzer model 1512: for creatinine the method of *Folin and Wu,* modified by *Hawk* et al. [14] and for uric acid the method of *Lofland and Crouse* [15].

(2) Optica Spectrophotometer model CF4: for glucose the enzymatic method [16] using the Boeringer kit; for urea the method of *Watt and Chrisp* [17]; for vitamin B_{12} the method of US Pharmacopeia [18]; for phenobarbital the UV method [19]; for salicylate the Pierce rapid stat kit, a modification of the Trinder method [20], and for inulin the anthrone method [21].

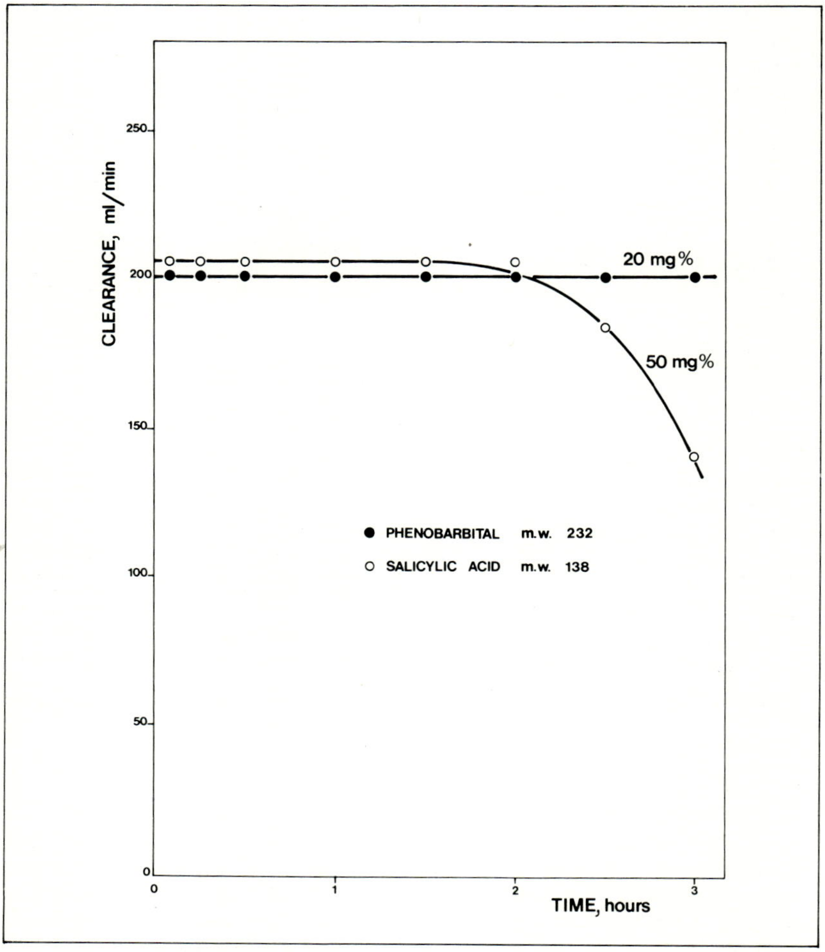

Fig. 6. Phenobarbital and salicylic acid clearances vs. time for two detoxyl 2 columns in series.

Results

Figure 5–7 show the in vitro clearances as function of perfusion time for the test substances. Figures 8 and 9 show the absorption isotherms for the uncoated carbon column respectively for creatinine and inulin. Table I shows the results of Coulter counter analysis of inlet and effluents of 13 uncoated and 13 cellulose-coated carbon columns.

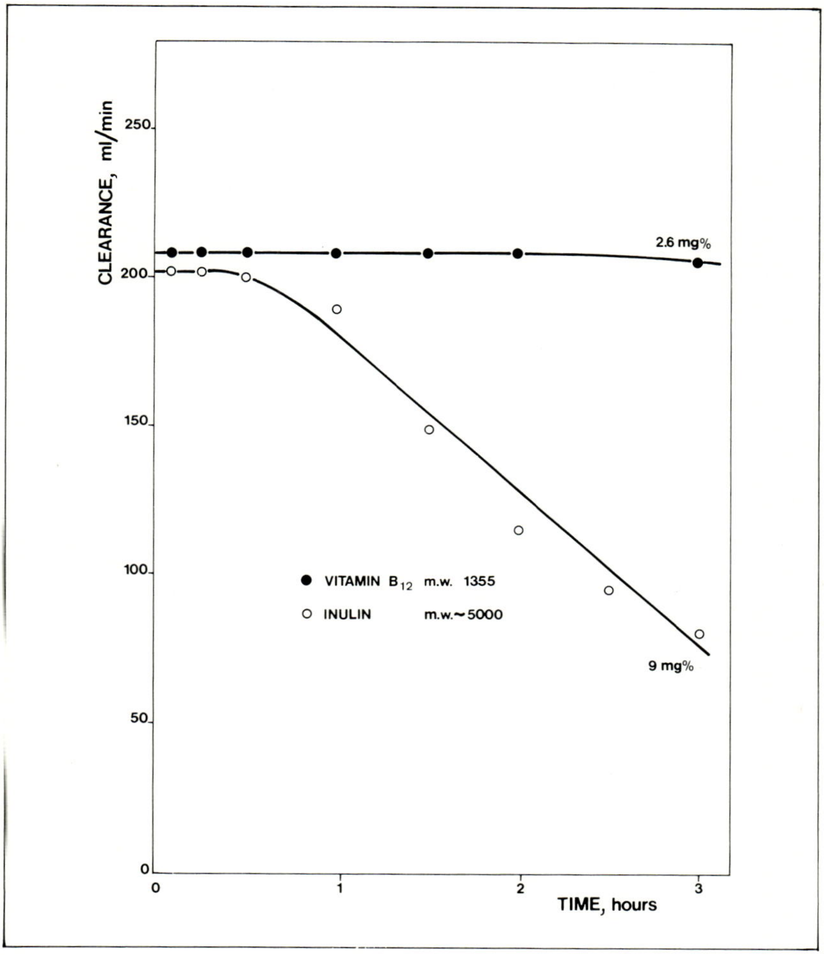

Fig. 7. Vitamin B_{12} and inulin clearances vs. time for two detoxyl 2 columns in series.

Discussion

The main purpose in the treatment of acute poisoning is the fast removal of the poison from body tissues. In this condition the use of a device characterized by high adsorption capacity and small priming volume, is very desirable. Figure 2 clearly shows that the coating deeply reduces the adsorption rate and capacity of the activated carbon particularly for medium and high molecular weight sub-

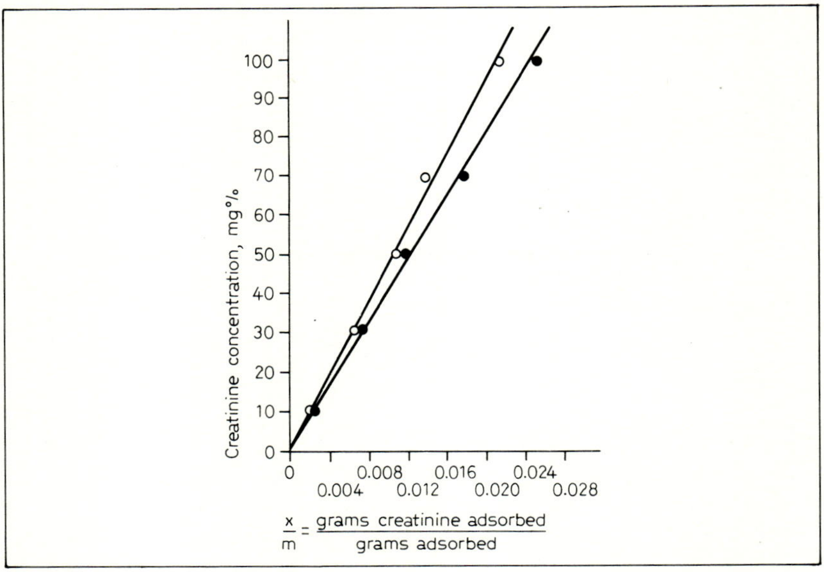

Fig. 8. Creatinine (mol. wt. 113) adsorption isotherms for uncoated (•) and (○) cellulose-coated activated carbon.

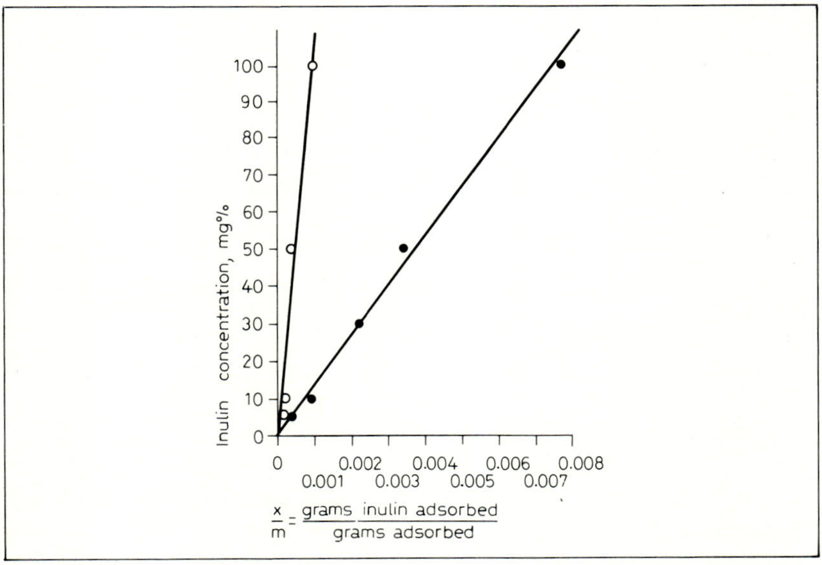

Fig. 9. Inulin (mol. wt. ~5,000) adsorption isotherms for uncoated (•) and (○) cellulose-coated activated carbon.

Table I. Microparticles determination in uncoated and cellulose-coated column effluent (average data of 13 columns of each type)

Device tested		Number of microparticles: Particle size dimension range		
		1,8–5 μm	5–10 μm	10–25 μm
Uncoated carbon	(inlet)	641 ± 10	20 ± 3	7 ± 2
	(1 liter effluent)	550 ± 12	21 ± 4	7 ± 2
Coated carbon	(inlet)	565 ± 15	19 ± 4	10 ± 2
	(1 liter effluent)	374 ± 20	17 ± 3	12 ± 5

stances. The same phenomenon is clearly illustrated by the adsorption isotherms (fig. 8, 9) for creatinine and inulin. In the case of creatinine (molec. wt. 113) the adsorption isotherms for uncoated and cellulose-coated activated carbon are only slightly different but for inulin (mol. wt. 5,000) the adsorption isotherms are very different due to the resistance of the membrane to inulin diffusion. The in vitro clearance data (fig. 5–7) show excellent adsorption characteristics of the column, especially taking into mind, that the amount of activated carbon contained in each column is only 80 g. The clearance for phenobarbital equals the perfusion flow rate after 3 h of hemoperfusion. In the case of salicylic acid, the columns (two in series) saturation starts only after 2 h of hemoperfusion during which the clearance was almost equal to the flow rate.

The microparticles generation rate of the columns prepared as described is shown in table I. The results confirm that the use of inherently hard carbon with regular shape immobilized in an appropriate column, makes practically insignificant the particles release also utilizing a sensitive measuring method as Coulter counting. It is important to stress that these results, significantly better than those reported by *Otsubo* et al. [22] with similar activated carbons, are deeply influenced by the column manufacturing technology, geometry and particularly by the column washing procedure. A deep pulsing of flow, during the washing, is able to mobilize and strip away the dust microparticles not previously removed during carbon washing.

In conclusion the microparticle generation from a hemoperfusion column could be controlled through an appropriate manufacturing and washing procedure utilizing an intrinsically hard and regularly shaped activated carbon, without coating. This type of device characterized by high adsorption capacity for a wide range of molecules could be advantageously used in acute poisoning.

Summary

In acute poisoning the main purpose of any therapeutic approach is a rapid removal of the drug or poison from body tissues. This approach suggested to undertake a study for the development of an uncoated activated carbon hemoperfusion column suitable for acute poisoning. The clearances were significantly superior compared with a similar device manufactured using coated carbon. The microparticle generation, utilizing a spherical type of activated carbon, was undetectable with the adopted measuring method, well below the US and British Pharmacopeas limits and practically equal to a coated carbon column with identical geometry.

References

1 Yatzidis, H.: A convenient hemoperfusion microapparatus over charcoal for the treatment of endogenous and exogenous intoxications: its use as an effective artificial kidney. Proc. Eur. Dial. Transplant. Ass. *1:* 83–87 (1964).
2 Dunea, G.; Kolff, W.J.: Clinical experience with the Yatzidis charcoal artificial kidney. Trans. Am. Soc. artif. internal Organs *11:* 178–182 (1965).
3 Hagstam, K.E.; Larsson, L.E.; Thysell, H.: Acta med. scand. *180:* 593–603 (1966).
4 Hagstam, K.E.; Larsson, L.E.; Thysell, H.: Proc. Eur. Dial. Transplant. Ass. *3:* 352–354 (1966).
5 Chang, T.M.S.: Artificial cells (Thomas, Springfield 1972).
6 Chang, T.M.S.: Protective effects of microencapsulation (coating) on platelet depletion and particulate embolism in the clinical applications of charcoal haemoperfusion: in Artificial organs. Strathclyde Bioengineering Seminars, chap. 19 (Macmillan, New York 1977).
7 Andrade, J.D.; Van Wagenen, R.; Chen, C.; Kopp, K.; Kolff, W.J.: Activated carbon and blood perfusion. Proc. Eur. Dial. Transplant. Ass. *9:* 21 (1972).
8 Denti, E.; Walker, J.M.; Luboz, M.P.; Tessore, V.; Malinverni, A.: Hemocompatibility problems in blood detoxification by activated carbon. Proc. Eur. Soc. artif. Organs *2:* 215 (1975).
9 Denti, E.; Luboz, M.P.; Tessore, V.: Adsorption characteristics of cellulose acetate coated charcoals. J. Biomed. Mater. Res. *9:* 143–150 (1975).
10 Gilchrist, T.; Johnson, E.; Martin, A.M.; Naucler, L.; Cameron, A.: Artificial liver support; pp. 319–328 (Williams Murray-Lyon) (Pitman, London 1975).
11 Fennimore, J.; Munro, G.D.: Artificial liver support, pp. 330–336 (Williams Murray-Lyon) (Pitman, London 1975).
12 Hill, J.B.; Palaia, F.L.; Horres, C.R.: The design of a charcoal haemoperfusion system; in Artificial organs. Strathclyde Bioengineering Seminars, chap. 14 (Macmillan, New York 1977).
13 Denti, E.; Walker, J.M.: Activated carbon: properties, selection, and evaluation in sorbents and their clinical applications, chap. 5, pp. 101–116 (Academic Press, New York 1980).
14 Hawk; Oser; Simmerson: Practical physiological chemistry; 12th ed., p. 506 (Blakiston, Philadelphia 1966).
15 Lofland, H.B.; Crouse, L.: Tech. Symp. *1:* 356 (1966–1967).
16 Werner, W.; Ray, H.G.; Wielinger, H.: Z. analyt. Chem. *252:* 224 (1970).
17 Watt, G.W.; Chrisp, J.D.: Analyt. Chem. *26:* 452–453 (1954).

18 US Pharmacopeia XIX, July 1, p. 110 (1975).
19 Frankel, S.; Reitman, S.; Sonnenwirth, A.C.: Clinical laboratory methods and diagnosis; 1st ed., pp. 343–344 (Mosby, Saint Louis 1970).
20 Macdonald, R.P.: Standard methods of clinical chemistry, vol. 5, pp. 405–409 (Academic Press, New York 1965).
21 Richterich, R.: Chimica clinica; teoria e pratica, pp. 392–394 (Bulzoni, Rome 1968).
22 Otsubo, O.; Horinchi, T.; Uchima, T.; Takai, N.; Tsunetsugu, T.; Inou, T.: Direct hemoperfusion with noncoated charcoal of high adsorption capacity derived from thermosetting resin. Trans. Am. Soc. artif. internal Organs *26:* 124–128 (1980).

V. Tessore, MD, Sorin Biomedica S.p.A., I–13040 Saluggia (Italy)

Contr. Nephrol., vol. 29, pp. 76–81 (Karger, Basel 1982)

Removal of Alpha-Amanitin from Blood by Hemoperfusion over Uncoated Charcoal

Experimental Results[1]

E. Masini, P. Blandina, P.F. Mannaioni

Department of Pharmacology and Toxicology, University of Florence, Italy

Introduction

In clinical toxicology, charcoal hemoperfusion is already an established device for shortening the half-life of drugs which cause severe intoxications. Its use should be restricted to the most serious life-threatening situations, for example, in the case of barbiturate overdose and of *Amanita phalloides* (verna, virosa) poisoning, which accounts for 7.8 and 11.1% of deaths, respectively [1].

Uncoated charcoal hemoperfusion (Detoxil-2 Sorin Biomedica, Saluggia, Italy) has been shown to be capable of combining high adsorption capability with a good blood compatibility leading to a quick and uneventful recovery from severe barbiturate poisoning; the clearance values were higher than those obtained with coated charcoal columns in similar clinical conditions [2, 3]. As far as *Amanita phalloides* poisoning is concerned, the clinical efficacy of charcoal hemoperfusion and the removal rate of mushroom toxins under experimental conditions have recently been evaluated.

Poisoned patients have been successfully treated with charcoal hemoperfusion [4–8] without apparent side effects. Labelled and unlabelled toxic peptides from *A. phalloides* have been efficiently removed from aqueous or plasma protein solution by charcoal perfusion in vitro [9, 10] and in phalloidin-intoxicated rats. Charcoal hemoperfusion allows a considerable increase in [^{14}C]-methyl phalloidin elimination, but is not accompanied by any significant prolongation of the survival period [11].

[1] Supported by a grant from National Research Council, Special Programme on Biomedical Technology, Subproject Farm 3.

α-Amanitin is recognised as the main offender in fatal human Amanita intoxications [12], and definite evidence for α-amanitin binding to uncoated activated charcoal is still lacking. Therefore, in the present study we report the results of experiments on the use of hemoperfusion for the therapy of acute clinical poisoning.

Material and Methods

α-Amanitin (Boehringer Mannheim, GmbH) was added to fresh heparinised human blood (250 ml) in concentrations ranging from 50–1,000 ng · ml^{-1}. The amanitin-containing blood was recirculated for 30 min using a hemoperfusion circuit similar to that employed in clinical hemoperfusion. The circuit was made up for an LKB roller pump to produce an upward flow through a Detoxyl 2 column at 200 ml/min and a manometer and a bubble trap. The column contains about 80 g of sorbent with a priming volume of 70 ± 5 ml. The characteristics of the charcoal and the geometry of the column have been described elsewhere [13]. At the end of the hemoperfusion (30 min) the column was disconnected from the perfusion lines and carefully washed with 250 ml of saline to remove loosely bound α-amanitin. The washed column was then eluted with 250 ml of 0.1 *N* HCl to remove tightly bound α-amanitin.

The concentration of α-amanitin present in the saline washings and in the acid eluates was evaluated by means of a radioimmunoassay described by *Faulstich* [12]. The method uses rabbit antiamanitin antibodies of the IgG class, which have been covalently attached to the nylon surface of a small nylon net. The IgG antibodies have been complexed with tritium labelled amatoxin to five fixed beads [^{3}H] antigen antibodies complexes. The nylon net was incubated for 2 h in the saline washings and in the acid eluates to be assayed. When incubated in the presence of amatoxins the radioactively labelled toxin will be released into the solute, and the radioactivity is counted in a Packard Tricarb (model 460 C). The method allows the detection of α-amanitin at the minimal concentration of 3 ng · ml^{-1}. The reproducibility of the method was checked in a clinical case of *A. phalloides* poisoning in a 61-year-old female patient at the fourth day of hospitalisation. She was on penicilin G therapy (40 · 10^6 IU/day). Her urinary concentration of α-amanitin was 8 ng · ml^{-1}, accounting for a total daily excretion of 13.6 μg and an excretion of 566 ng/h. Similar values of urinary excretion of α-amanitin in 2 cases of clinical poisoning have been recently reported by *Costantino* et al. [14], using the radioimmunoassay described by *Fiume* et al. [15].

Results

Hemoperfusion of blood containing α-amanitin through a Detoxyl 2 column for 30 min results in a satisfactory binding of α-amanitin to uncoated activated charcoal. The following results were obtained in analysing the column which has been used for 30 min of hemoperfusion. No α-amanitin was eluted by saline. However, α-amanitin was eluted by acid and the amount of α-amanitin recovered in the acid eluates showed a linear relationship with the amanitin blood levels (fig. 1).

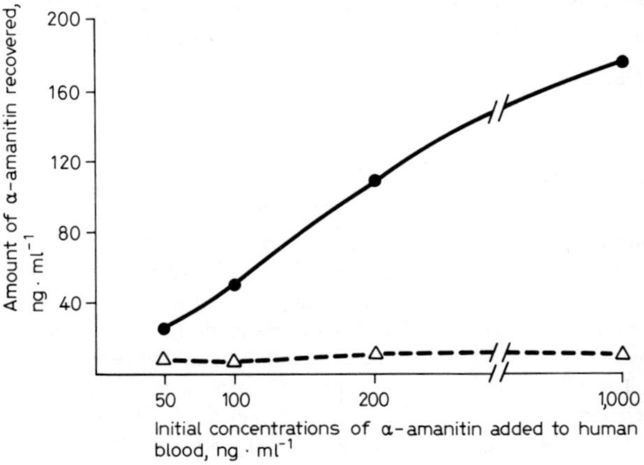

1

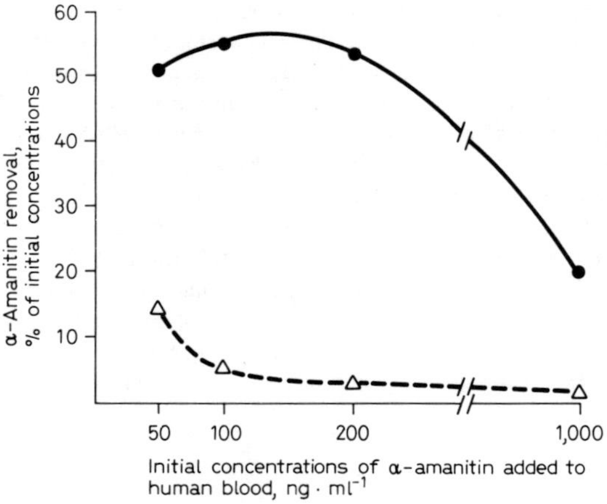

2

Fig. 1, 2. Removal of α-amanitin from human blood by a Detoxyl-2 column. ● = acid eluates; △ = saline washings. Each point represents triplicate assays from four separate experiments.

Table I. Removal of amanitin from human blood by a Detoxyl-2 column[1]

Experiment No.	α-Amanitin added		α-Amanitin in acid eluates		%
	ng · ml⁻¹	μg total	ng · ml⁻¹	μg total	removed
1	50	12	26	6.70	52
2	100	25	55	13.75	55
3	200	50	110	27.50	55
4	1,000	250	178	44.50	18

[1] 30 min hemoperfusion, 1 Detoxyl-2 column (80 g).

As shown in figure 2, the removal of α-amanitin from human blood by a Detoxyl 2 column is a function of the initial concentration of α-amanitin in the blood. A steady removal ranging from 50 to 60% of the initial concentration was achieved with blood amanitin levels between 50 and 200 ng · ml^{-1}; a sharp decrease of amanitin removal was observed at blood amanitin concentrations between 200 and 1,000 ng · ml^{-1}. The results are summarized in table I, which stresses the good adsorption capacity of uncoated activated charcoal toward α-amanitin, especially in the range of the lower blood amanitin levels.

Discussion

Seeger and Bartels [9] have shown that perfusion in vitro over acrylic hydrogel-coated charcoal resulted in almost complete detoxication of an extract of *A. phalloides* in aqueous or plasma protein solutions; similar results have been reported by *Langenscheid* et al. [10] using hemoperfusion over polymeric adsorbents. Our present experiments confirm these data, and also indicate a good sorbent capability for α-amanitin by uncoated activated charcoal. In experiments using Detoxyl 2 columns, it has been shown [16] that plasma albumins produce a physiological coating of carbon microparticles in a simple pass through the carbon surfaces. Since it is widely accepted [17] that α-amanitin is bound to plasma albumin, the coating by α-amanitin albumin complexes of the uncoated carbon microparticles could also be accounted for by the high adsorption rate observed in our experiments. The exhaustion of the sorbent capability of Detoxyl 2 columns toward high α-aminitin blood levels is easily explained in terms of saturation of binding sites.

Despite the good adsorption capability of coated or uncoated activated charcoal toward mushroom toxins, it is still hard to say how much clinical hemoperfusion should be useful in the clinical management of *A. phalloides* poisoning. In considering this possibility it should be kept in mind that the plasma levels of α-amanitin so far recorded in clinical poisonings are far below the levels used in experiments dealing with the evaluation of the absorption rate (ranging from 1 to 24 ng · ml^{-1}) [14, 18] and in some cases undetectable even after 11–13 h from the ingestion of toxic mushrooms [18]. These low concentrations of α-amanitin in the blood (in contrast with the good elimination of α-amanitin in the urine) [14] may suggest that mushroom toxins have a high distribution volume, a condition which is known to hamper any procedure of blood purification.

In conclusion, the routine application of charcoal hemoperfusion in clinical *A. phalloides* poisoning must await further information about the toxicokinetics of mushroom toxins in intoxicated patients, and should be restricted only to those patients in which suitable blood α-amanitin levels have been detected. This caution is also stressed by the fact that hemoperfusion could influence, unfavorably, the coagulation pattern which is already unbalanced by the hepatotoxicity of mushroom toxins.

Summary

The sorbent capacity of uncoated charcoal column (Detoxyl 2, Sorin Biomedica) on α-amanitin was studied by adding known amounts of α-amanitin to fresh human blood, which was recirculated through a clinical hemoperfusion circuit over a period of 30 min. The column was washed with saline to remove loosely bound α-amanitin, and eluted with 0.1 *N* HCl to detach absorbed α-amanitin. α-amanitin concentration was measured in the saline washings and in the acid eluates by means of a radioimmunoassay. Only negligible amounts of amanitin were recovered in the saline washings. Suitable amounts of α-amanitin were present in the acid eluates, showing an adsorption optimum for blood concentrations ranging from 50 to 200 ng · ml^{-1}. The results were discussed as predictable of the clinical usefulness of charcoal hemoperfusion in *A. phalloides* poisoning.

References

1 Mannaioni, P.F.: Le intossicazioni Acute; in Teodori, Manuale di Terapia Medica (Società Editrice Universo, Roma, in press).

2 Martinelli, R.; Sodi, A.; Denti, E.; Walker, J.; Mannaioni, P.F.: Charcoal hemoperfusion for acute drug intoxication. Case reports; in Sideman, Chang, Hemoperfusion, kidney and liver support and intoxication, pp. 307–318 (Hemisphere Publishing, Washington 1980).

3 Fantozzi, R.; Martinelli, R.; Masini, E.; Sodi, A.; Amaducci, L.; Mannaioni, P.F.: Management of acute intoxications with barbiturate and salicylate by uncoated charcoal hemoperfusion. Substance Alcohol Action/Misuse. *2:* 55–62, 1981.

4 Bartels, O.; Grumeth, M.; Daniel, U.; Haas, T.D.; Kramer, G.; Tympener, R.: Frühzeitige Kohlehämoperfusion bei Knollenblätter-Pilzvergiftung. Dt. med. Wschr. *100:* 2509 (1975).

5 Okonek, S.: Hemoperfusion with coated activated charcoal for treating acute poisoning by remidies, plant protectant and fungi. Medsche Klin. *71:* 1120–1122 (1976).
6 Okonek, S.: Hemoperfusion with coated activated charcoal for treating acute poisoning by remedies, plant protectans and fungi. Medsche Klin. *72:* 862–866 (1977).
7 Denti, E.; Triolo, R.; Grivet, V.; Ramello, A.: Charcoal hemoperfusion in mushroom poisoning *Amanita phalloides;* in Chang, Artificial liver, artificial kidney, artificial cells (Plenum Press, New York 1978).
8 Wauters, J.P.; Rossel, C.; Farquet, J.J.: *Amanita phalloides* poisoning treated by charcoal hemoperfusion. Br. med. J. *ii:* 1465–1470 (1978).
9 Seeger, R.; Bartels, O.: The elimination of toxic peptides from *Amanita phalloides* by charcoal hemoperfusion in vitro. Dt. med. Wschr. *101:* 1456–1459 (1976).
10 Langenscheid, C.; Schimitz-Salve, H.; Faulstich, H.; Kramer, P.; Scheler, R.: In vitro elimination or [^{3}H]-methyl-dehydroxymethyl α-amanitin by four extracorporeal purification methods; in Faulstich, Kommierell, Wieland, Amanita toxins and amanita poisoning (Witzrock, New York, in press).
11 Rockel, A.; Schmid, G.; Rupp, P.; Kult, J.; Hennemann, H.; Heidland, A.: Hämoperfusion mit Aktivkohle und Ionenaustauscher bei Phalloides-vergifteten Ratten. Dt. med. Wschr *101:* 418–420 (1976).
12 Faulstich, H.: New aspects of amanita poisoning. Klin. Wschr. *57:* 1143–1152 (1979).
13 Tessore, V.; Luboz, M.P.; Denti, E.: The use of uncoated activated carbon hemoperfusion in acute poisoning. In vitro studies. This issue.
14 Costantino, D.; Brega, A.; Langer, M.; Fiume, L.; Gavazzeni, V.; Vesconi, S.; Busi, C.; Iapichino, C.; Rivolta, E.: Contributo allo studio della cinetica della amanita nell'uomo. Anest. Rianimazione *18:* 267–274 (1977).
15 Fiume, L.; Busi, C.; Campadelli-Fiume, G.; Franceschi, C.: Production of antibodies to amanitin as the basis for their radioimmunoassay. Experientia *31:* 1233 (1975).
16 Denti, E.; Walker, J.M.: in Sorbents and their clinical application, chap. 5, pp. 101–116 (Academic Press, New York 1980).
17 Floersheim, G.: in Faulstich, Kommerell, Wieland, Chemotherapy of amanita poisoning (Witzrock, New York, in press).
18 Busi, C.; Fiume, L.; Costantino, D.; Borroni, M.; Ambrosino, G.; Olivotto, A.; Bernardini, D.: Détermination des amanitines dans le serum de patients intoxiqués par l'*Amanite phalloide.* Nouv. Presse méd. *6:* 2855–2857 (1977).

E. Masini, MD, Department of Pharmacology and Toxicology, University of Florence, I–50100 Florence (Italy)

Contr. Nephrol., vol. 29, pp. 82–89 (Karger, Basel 1982)

Hemoperfusion in Diabetic Coma

C. Giordano, R. Esposito, P. Bello, E. Quarto, D. Cirillo, M. Pluvio, N. Lanzetti, L. Calabria

Chair of Nephrology, 1st Faculty of Medicine, University of Naples, Naples, Italy

Introduction

Hemoperfusion is an elective treatment for several types of endogenous and exogenous intoxications. In fact, its application is useful in cases of abnormal ingestion of drugs and toxins [1–4] and in some cases of severe failure of organs, i.e. hepatic coma [5–8] or uremia [8, 9]. The sorbent commonly used in this technique is active carbon in a coated or uncoated form. However, it has no success when it is necessary for electrolyte management. In these cases ion-exchange resins can be used either for removal of anions and cations, or for acid base balance re-equilibration [10–14].

In this work the use of the hemoperfusion technique on anionic resins for diabetic keto-acidosis (DKA) coma is proposed. The DKA coma, which still has a 6–9% fatal outcome alone or together with other complications [15, 16], is in fact characterized by a 30-fold increase of keto acids, a fall of bicarbonate to 10–5 mEq/l, and a fall of blood pH down to 6.9–7.0.

Hemoperfusion was performed utilizing a strong anionic exchange resin in the mixed form (HCO_3^- and Cl^- form), which is able to exchange the increased ketoanions and organic anions against bicarbonate in a stoichiometric manner, giving this to patients in a smooth physiological fashion. This technique represents a useful advantage in respect to the therapy with bicarbonate infusion, where the administration is abrupt with a consequent possible rise of hypokalemia and tissue hypoxia [17]. In addition, in the latter case there was no removal of ketoanions from the patients.

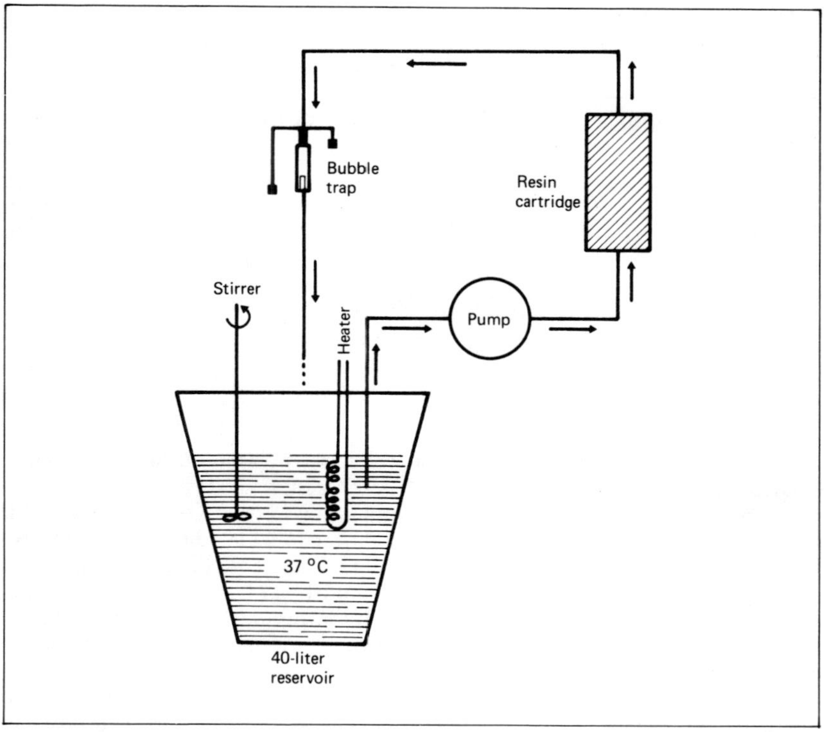

Fig. 1. Simulated hemoperfusion apparatus.

Material and Methods

The resin utilized is a strong anionic resin, A_{500} Kastel Montedison, with the following characteristics: shipping density 0.73 kg/l; effective density 1.07 kg/l; moisture 50%; total exchange capacity 1,200 mEq/l of humid resin and 3,300 mEq/kg of dry resin. The resin was used in bicarbonate-chloride mixed form and was obtained through mixing in the desired proportions of resin in the HCO_3^- form and of resin in the Cl^- form. The resin in the HCO_3^- form was prepared with a treatment of excess of $NaHCO_3$ 5% solution (15 l/kg humid resin with a flow rate of 250 ml/min); afterwards it was washed with distilled water until elimination of $NaHCO_3$. Similarly the resin in chloride form was prepared with a treatment of excess of NaCl 5% solution (10 l/kg humid resin; flow rate 250 ml/min); afterwards it was washed with distilled water until elimination of NaCl. The mixtures of resins utilized were, respectively, 6% HCO_3^- – 94% Cl^-, 9% HCO_3^- – 91% Cl^- and 15% HCO_3^- – 85% Cl^-. The trials on the resins were made in open circuit to determine the characteristics of exchange per unit weight of resin, and in closed circuit in order to simulate hemoperfusion.

Table I. Experimental conditions in simulated hemoperfusion

	Simulated hemoperfusion		
Cartridge	Resin A500 (9% HCO_3^- and 91% Cl^- from) weight 1,700 g		
Patient	40 ± 2 liters	Cl^-	102.0 ± 0.5 mEq/l
		HCO_3^-	10.3 ± 0.2 mEq/l
		Ketoanions	26.5 ± 0.5 mEq/l
		Lactate	3.01 ± 0.05 mEq/l
Flow rate	200 ± 25 ml/min		
Time	4 h.		

Open circuit trials were performed processing the resins in the indicated amount with solutions of the following composition: (a) 55 g of dry resin (15% HCO_3^- form): [Cl^-] = 102.5 mEq/l; [HCO_3^-] = 20.2 mEq/l; [ketoanions] ([acetoacetate] = 12.1 mEq/l and [β-hydroxybutyrate] = 7.0 mEq/l) = 19.1 mEq/l; flow rate 23 ml/min. (b) 50 g of dry resin (9% HCO_3^- form): [Cl^-] = 101.0 mEq/l; [HCO_3^-] = 20.1 mEq/l; [ketoanions ([acetoacetate] = 11.9 mEq/l and [β-hydroxybutyrate] = 7.1 mEq/l)] = 19.0 mEq/l; [lactate] = 3.0 mEq/l; flow rate 25 ml/min. (c) 46 g of dry resin (6% HCO_3^- form): [Cl^-] = 103.0 mEq/l; [HCO_3^-] = 20.5 mEq/l; [ketoanions] ([acetoacetate] = 12 mEq/l and [β-hydroxybutyrate] = 7.3 mEq/l) = 19.3 mEq/l; flow rate 22 ml/min.

These resins are put in short columns (length:diameter ratio 1:2.5) to reduce HCO_3^- concentration peaks in effluent liquids [14]. A flow speed of 2 m/h inside the columns was obtained. Closed circuit trials were performed using resin cartridges 14 cm in diameter and 33 cm in length. Experiments were performed using the apparatus reported in figure 1. From a 40-liter reservoir simulating a 70-kg patient, the fluid goes through a cartridge containing 1.7 kg of the resin 9% HCO_3^- form. Pressure drop in cartridge was always inferior to 0.20–0.25 H_2O meter. Flow rate was about 200 ml/min. No liquid filled the resin bed before hemoperfusion trials; in such a way the osmolality of processed fluid was constant. The main experimental conditions are reported in table I.

Anion concentrations were detected with the following methods: (1) Chloride using the Mohr method. (2) Ketoanions (β-hydroxybutyrate and acetoacetate) transforming with hydroxybutyrate-dehydrogenase the β-hydroxybutyrate to acetoacetate and detecting thereafter the acetone, obtained from thermic decomposition from acetoacetate gas chromatography [18]. (3) Lactate was determined by enzymatic methods using lactate dehydrogenase [19, 20]. (4) Bicarbonate by gas volumetric method [21].

Results

Open Circuit Trials

These experiments were performed to determine either the amount of milliequivalents exchanged on the resins, or the behavior of anions in liquids processed on the resins in different percentages of the HCO_3^- form.

Table II shows the amount of HCO_3^- milliequivalents released by resins in a working range of 30 liters/kg dry weight, the maximum HCO_3^- concentration in the effluent fluid, and the entrapped ketoanions milliequivalents. It can be noticed that the amount of entrapped ketoanions is almost constant in all cases for all resins; instead, the amount of released HCO_3^- and the maximum concentration of this ion increase in a nonproportional manner in regard to the rise of the percentage of the HCO_3^- form. The resin in the 9% HCO_3^- form presents a peak of 38 mEq/l and a high enough release of bicarbonate (235 mEq). For these reasons the latter resin is chosen for hemoperfusion application.

The behavior of the anions in the fluid leaving the resin 9% HCO_3^- form is reported in figure 2. The shaded areas represent the milliequivalents released or trapped on 50 g of resin in a 1.5 liter working range. In this figure the lactate behavior is also reported; the HCO_3^- concentration ranges in the almost physiological limits.

Table III shows the anion exchanges relative to the 1 kg of dry resin 9% HCO_3^- form: a release of 235 mEq of bicarbonates happens together with a trapping of either 188 mEq ketoanions or 14 mEq lactate.

Simulated Hemoperfusion Trials

Data obtained in open circuit experiments indicate the best conditions to perform experiments in closed circuit systems. In table IV the mean values obtained in 10 'hemoperfusions' according to the previously indicated conditions are reported. The fluid was recirculated for 4 h on the 1.7 kg of resin 9% HCO_3^- form. The data concerning the anion balance in the 40-liter reservoir are also listed in the table: an HCO_3^- exchange of 400 mEq occurs against 344 mEq of ketoanions and lactate (86%) and only 56 mEq of Cl^- (14%). In such a way a 30% removal of ketoanion is obtained and the HCO_3^- concentration is doubled. In figure 3 a typical anion behavior is reported in a simulated hemoperfusion. After 2 h, at a flow rate of 200 ml/min, the greatest part of resin is exhausted and anion concentrations approximate the asymptomatic values. For in vivo experiments, it is better to reduce to a half or a quarter of the above flow rate, prolonging the hemoperfusion time for 4 or 8 h. This means a more physiological approach of HCO_3^- administration to the patient.

Discussion

Results in open and in closed circuits show a satisfactory removal of ketoanions and a simultaneous release of bicarbonates in a physiological manner. This is obtained utilizing a moderate amount of resin and in a satisfactory amount of time. This means that in an in vivo experiment, utilizing a 50–100 ml/min blood flow rate, it is possible to double HCO_3^- concentration in 4–6 h and

Table II. Bicarbonates and ketoanions released or trapped on A500 resin in different HCO_3^- form

Anion	% of resin in HCO_3^- form	Dry resin released (+) or trapped (–), mEq/kg	HCO_3^- concentration maximum, mEq/l
	15	+306	60
HCO_3^-	9	+235	38
	6	+45	26
	15	–196	
Ketoanions	9	–188	
	6	–183	

Table III. Milliequivalents of ions released or trapped per kilogram of resin A500 9% HCO_3^- form

Anion	Inlet concentration, mEq/l	Dry resin released (+) or trapped (–), mEq/l
Cl^-	104.0	–33
HCO_3^-	20.0	+235
Acetoacetate	11.9	–188
β-Hydroxybutyrate	7.1	
Lactate	3.0	–14

Table IV. Mean ion values of ten simulated hemoperfusions: 4 h hemoperfusion on 1.7 kg of A500 resin in mixed form (9% HCO_3^- and 91% Cl^-)

Anion	Initial concentration, mEq/l	Final concentration, mEq/l	Reservoir balance, mEq/l
Cl^-	102.0 ± 0.5	100.4 ± 0.5	–56 ± 20
HCO_3^-	10.3 ± 0.5	20.3 ± 0.5	+400 ± 20
Ketoanions	26.5 ± 0.5	18.5 ± 0.5	–320 ± 20
Lactate	3.01 ± 0.05	2.41 ± 0.05	–24 ± 2

to remove about 350 mEq of ketoanions and other organic anions in respect to the blood osmolality. At the same time, in this case the blood pH rises by 0.3, as can be deduced by doubling HCO_3^- in the Henderson-Hasselbach equation and keeping all other conditions unchanged. In such a way, a better utilization of insulin is obtained as this hormone is inhibited in acidic medium. At pH 7 only 60–70% of the original activity of insulin is retained and the activity falls rapidly as the pH continues to decrease. As the pH increases towards normal, glucose

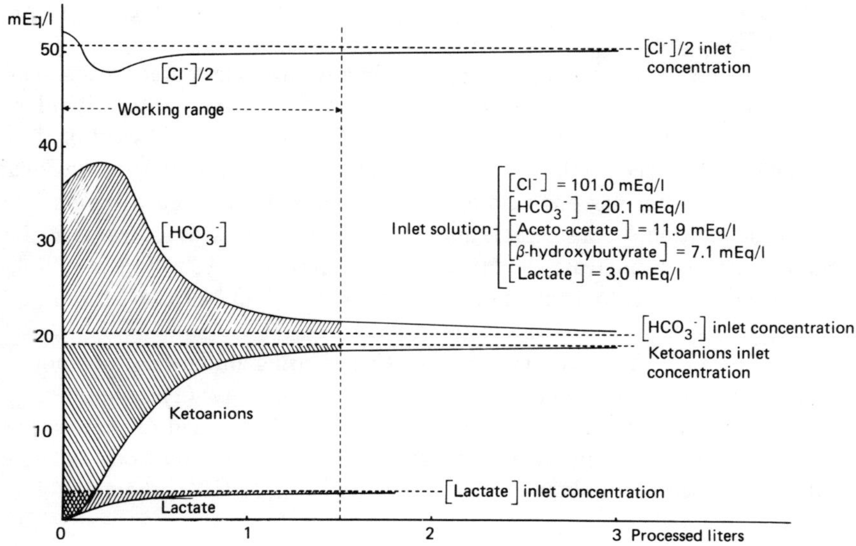

Fig. 2. Cl^-, HCO_3^-, lactate and ketoanions on 50 g of A500 strong anionic resin in mixed form (9% HCO_3^-, 91% Cl^- form). Flow rate 25 ml/min.

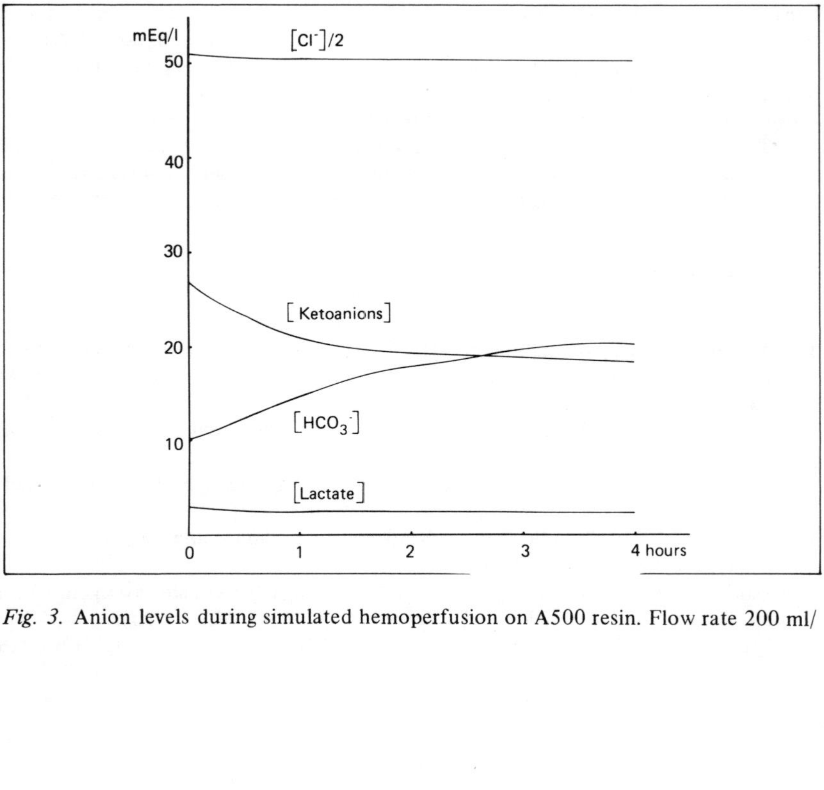

Fig. 3. Anion levels during simulated hemoperfusion on A500 resin. Flow rate 200 ml/min.

metabolism improves and ketoanion production decreases, resulting in improvement in ketoacidosis.

DKA hemoperfusion treatment presents many advantages over the standard $NaHCO_3$ infusion therapy. In fact, $NaHCO_3$ infusion has potential complications because of the high concentrations of HCO_3^- in the infused solution. The main side effects recently listed by *Genuth* [17] are: (1) abrupt hyperkalemia; (2) increased central nervous system acidosis, and (3) decreased tissue oxygen delivery. In addition, a considerable amount of liquid is infused; for instance, 2.5 liters are needed to increase the HCO_3^- concentration by 10 mEq/l in a 70-kg patient utilizing an isotonic solution of $NaHCO_3$ (1,4% of $NaHCO_3$, 166 mEq/l of HCO_3^-).

All these side effects can be eliminated when using anionic resin hemoperfusion and two goals are obtained at the same time, namely: (1) a smooth infusion of bicarbonates occurs at suitable concentration levels, and (2) ketoanions and organic anions are subtracted through direct exchange against 86% or more of HCO_3^- released and no liquid or Na^+ is required as in $NaHCO_3$ therapy.

Summary

Hemoperfusion on ionic exchange resins in the therapy of diabetic keto-acidosis (DKA) coma is proposed. Resins used are strong anionic resins in mixed form able to release bicarbonates and to trap ketoanions and organic anions in a stoichiometric manner. A series of trials in open circuit are performed in order to search for a suitable mixture of resins and to establish the amounts of HCO_3^- and ketoanions respectively released or entrapped. Therefore, ten simulated hemoperfusions in closed circuit systems were performed, utilizing cartridges containing 1,700 g of mixed resin (9% HCO_3^- form and 91% Cl^- form).

The results indicate that all side effects of bicarbonate i.v. therapy of DKA coma are avoided because of the smooth HCO_3^- administration to the patient. Furthermore, a good removal of ketoanions and organic acids is obtained without changing the blood osmolality.

References

1 Yatzidis, H.: A convenient hemoperfusion micro-apparatus over charcoal for the treatment of endogenous and exogenous intoxications. Proc. Eur. Dial. Transplant. Ass. *1:* 83 (1964).

2 Chang, T.M.S.: Removal of endogenous and exogenous toxins by micro-encapsulated absorbent. Can. J. Physiol. Pharmacol. *47:* 1043 (1969).

3 Lorch, J.A.; Garella, S.: Hemoperfusion to treat intoxication. Ann. intern. Med. *91:* 301 (1979).

4 Rosenbaum, J.L.: Poisinings; in Sorbents and their clinical applications, pp. 451–466 (Academic Press, New York 1980).

5 Gazzard, B.G.; Portmann, B.A.; Weston, M.I.; Longley, P.G.; Murray-Lyon, I.M.; Dunlop, E.H.; Flax, H.; Mellon, P.J.; Record, C.O.; Ward, M.B.; Williams, R.: Charcoal hemoperfusion in the treatment of fulminant hepatic failure. Lancet *i:* 1301 (1974).

6 Gelfand, M.C.; Knepshield, J.H.; Cohan, S.; Ramirez, B.; Schreiner, G.E.: Treatment of hepatic coma with hemoperfusion through polyacrylamide hydrogel-coated charcoal. Kidney int. *10:* S239 (1976).
7 Silk, D.B.A.; Williams, R.: Sorbents in hepatic failure; in Sorbents and their clinical applications, pp. 415–450 (Academic Press, New York 1980).
8 Chang, T.M.S.: Hemoperfusion alone and in series with ultrafiltration or dialysis for uremia, poising and liver failure. Kidney int. *10:* S 305 (1976).
9 Gelfand, M.C.; Winchester, J.F.: Hemoperfusion results in uremia. Clin. Nephrol. *11:* 107 (1979).
10 Gordon, A.; Martin, R.: Ion exchanges and their clinical applications; in Sorbents and their clinical application, pp. 249–273 (Academic Press, New York 1980).
11 Giordano, C.; Esposito, R.; Bello, P.; Quarto, E.: A resin sorbent system for regeneration of peritoneal fluid for dialysis. Dialysis transplant *8*: 351 (1979).
12 Giordano, C.; Esposito, R.; Bello, P.; Quarto, E.; Pluvio, M.: Peritoneal dialysis belt. Int. J. artif. Organs *3:* 139 (1980).
13 Esposito, R.; Pluvio, M.; Bello, P.; Quarto, E.; Savoia, S.; Giordano, C.: Uso di polialdeidi per via orale e di un rene artificiale indossabile nel trattamento dell'uremia cronica. Minerva nefrol. *27:* 425 (1980).
14 Esposito, R.; Bello, P.; Quarto, E.; Pluvio, M.; Cirillo, D.; Lanzetti, N.; Giordano, C.: The feasibility of electrolytes management in closed circuit system. Abstr. 3rd Int. Conf. on Uremia, Capri 1980, p. 26.
15 Beigelman, P.M.: Severe diabetic ketoacidosis (diabetic coma): 482 episodes in 257 patients. Experience of three years. Diabetes *20:* 490 (1981).
16 Soler, N.G.; Fitzgerald, M.G.; Bennet, M.A.; Malius, J.M.: Intensive care in the management of diabetic ketoacidosis. Lancet *i:* 951 (1973).
17 Genuth, S.: Diabetic ketoacidosis in clinical diabetes: modern management, pp. 173–207 (Appleton Century Crofts, New York 1980).
18 Siegel, L.; Robin, N.; McDonald, L.J.: New approach to determination of total ketone bodies in serum. Clin. Chem. *23:* 46 (1977).
19 Olson, G.F.: Optimal conditions for the enzymatic determination of *L*-lactic acid. Clin. Chem. *8:* 1 (1962).
20 Hohorst, H.J.: *L*–(+)–Lactate determination with lactic dehydrogenase and DPN; in Bergmeyer, Methods of enzymatic analysis, p. 226 (Academic Press, New York 1963).
21 Natelson, S.: Routine use of ultramicromethods in the clinical laboratory. J. clin. Path. *21:* 1153 (1951).

C. Giordano, MD, Chair of Nephrology, 1st Faculty of Medicine,
University of Naples, I–80100 Naples (Italy)

Contr. Nephrol., vol. 29, pp. 90–100 (Karger, Basel 1982)

Resin Hemoperfusion for Unconjugated Bilirubin Removal

S. Sideman, L. Mor, M. Mihich, D. Mordohovich, S. Lupovich, J.M. Brandes, M. Zeltzer

Department of Biomedical Engineering and School of Medicine, Technion, Israel Institute of Technology, Haifa, Israel

Introduction

The application of *Chang's* [1] 'artificial cell' concept to render biocompatibility to *Yatzidis's* [2] charcoal hemoperfusion (HP) microapparatus, provided the impetus to the recent development of hemoperfusion as a clinical mode of operation. A non-specific adsorbent, activated charcoal (AC) removes a wide range of toxic and physiological substances from the blood [35].

Resins, which actually precede AC as adsorbents for the artificial kidney [3, 4], extend the application of HP for blood purification. *Rosenbaum* et al. [5] initiated the clinical utilization of an aromatic, nonionic Amberlite XAD-4 resin columns (Extracorporeal Medical Specialities Ltd.) that has a particular adsorptive attraction for lipid-soluble drugs and no appreciable adsorptive effect on blood glucose, electrolytes, plasma proteins or lipids. Studies of other resins and their relative importance as sorbents in the treatment of uremia, hepatic failure and acute intoxification have also been reported [6–14]. However, only XAD-4 is presently recommended for clinical detoxification of a wide range of toxic materials [7, 14].

The variety of potential surface properties of the resins provide the tool for selective removal of specific solutes, thus overcoming some of the defects of AC and extending the range of application of HP. Here, we demonstrate the application of a specific resin to remove the albumin-bound unconjugated bilirubin from the blood.

A partially functioning liver is usually unable to clear the body of bilirubin, a product of the catabolic breakdown of hemoglobin. Large concentrations of bilirubin in the blood have therefore been associated with hepatic failure [15], and with neurological brain damage (and death) of newborn babies suffering from hemolysing diseases. The attempts to develop a liver support system led to in vitro and in vivo studies of bilirubin removal by charcoal [16, 17], uncharged resins [5], ion exchangers [17–22] and albumin-conjugated agarose gel beads [15, 23].

Sideman et al. [24–27] and others [19, 23, 28] have suggested the application of HP for the removal of the unconjugated bilirubin which is responsible for kernicterus, morbidity and mortality of jaundiced newborn babies. Here, we report some aspects of our development of a HP column, containing a macroreticular ion exchange resin with a biocompatible coating, which is suitable for unconjugated bilirubin removal.

Coating the AC particles is required to eliminate fine particle release as well as to avoid platelet depletion during HP of the chronically ill (uremic) patients [1, 30]. Resin beads have but little fines and the bare XAD-4 resin affects a 30–40% decrease in the circulating platelet concentration. Although this depletion is considered safe for a single detoxification HP treatment, it may nevertheless be dangerous in a device supporting patients requiring repeated treatments or newborn babies.

To overcome the problem of platelet loss and thrombocytopenia, *Sideman* et al. [24, 31] and others [1, 29, 32] suggested that the resin particles be coated with a thin layer of a biocompatible material. Poly-HEMA, acrylic polymers as well as a cross-linked albumin coating on Dowex 1X2 were evaluated [31]. Physically absorbed albumin has been used to render biocompatibility in charcoal hemoperfusion as early as 1969 [30] and more recently to Amberlite XAD-7 [21, 22, 29].

Minimal heparinization is desired in order to avoid spontaneous bleeding as well as to prevent blood clotting during the extracoporeal blood treatment. Either whole blood clotting time or activated partial thromboplastin time (APTT) are usually sampled during the extracorporeal procedure [33]. The heparin is administered either continuously or in hourly doses. *Gotch and Keen* [34] suggested a pharmacokinetic model for a priori prediction of desired heparinization levels in high risk bleeding patients. Here, we report our preliminary attempts to adopt this procedure to the heparinization of baboons during HP.

Resin Selection and Preparation

A number of gel type and macroreticular type ion exchange resins were tested for their bilirubin binding capacity [25, 26]. The macroreticular resin appears to have the best adsorption capacity for unconjugated bilirubin.

The bilirubin adsorption curves and the plasma pH characteristics of the MR resin during in vitro adsorption are presented in figure 1. The OH^- form increases the plasma pH while the Cl^- and the lactate forms decrease the plasma pH. The HCO_3^- form is stable and seems to have a minute effect on the pH. The release of HCO_3^- ions to the solution hardly affects the plasma pH.

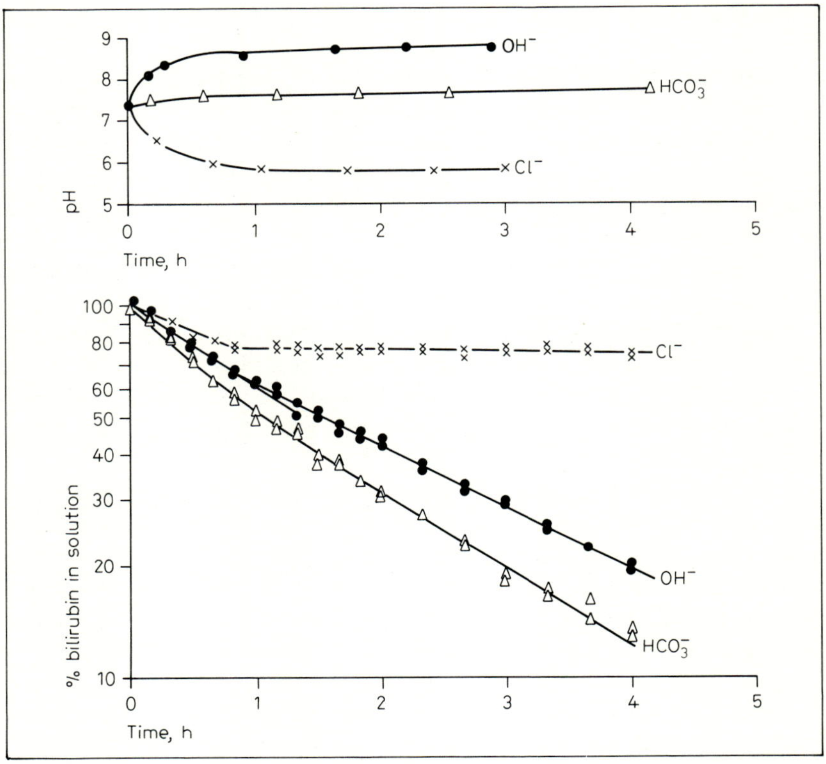

Fig. 1. pH and percent of the initial plasma unconjugated bilirubin concentration which remains during batch adsorption experiment. 20 ml bed volume of macroreticular resin shaken at 37 °C with 100 ml plasma containing 15 mg% unconjugated bilirubin.

As is well known, the adsorption of a weak acid like bilirubin on a weak base resin is limited to a narrow pH range, between the resin pK and the weak acid pK. In the Cl^- form of the MR resin, the solution pH decreases below pH = 6. Under these conditions the BIL is not ionized and its exchange with the ion exchanger will stop. In its OH^- form, the resin pH increases and approaches its pK, causing its exchange capacity to decrease. In the HCO_3^- form both the solution pH and the resin pH are at, or near, the optimum state and show a maximum BIL adsorption and minimum changes in the plasma pH.

The desired HCO_3^- ionic form was achieved by converting the previously conditioned resin to the Cl^- form, and then to the HCO_3^- form by 10 volumes of 1 *N* $NaHCO_3$.

The resin was coated with albumin by shaking a batch of resin particles in an albumin solution in PBS. The particles were then cross-linked by glutaral-

2 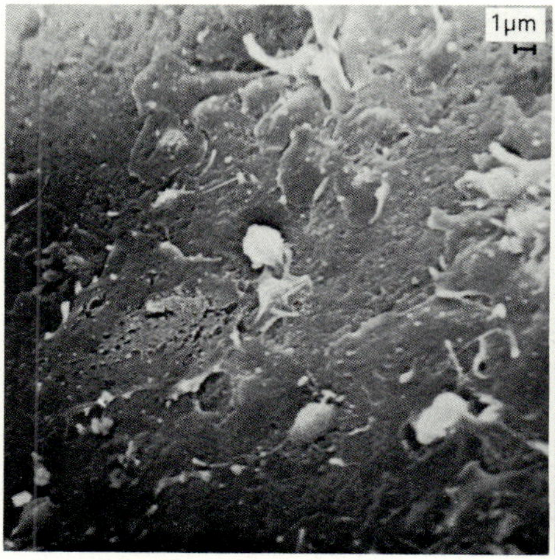

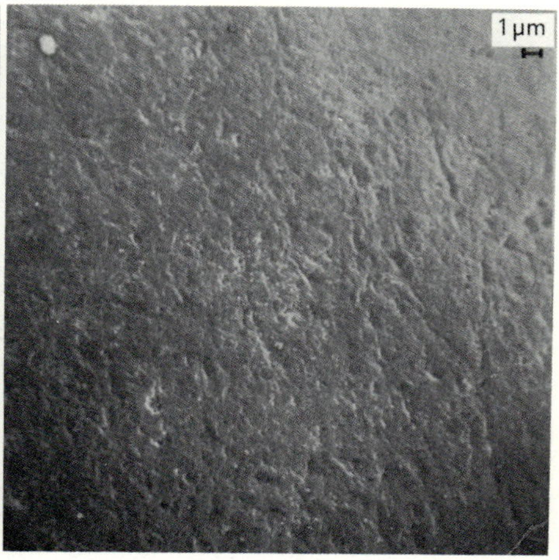 3

Fig. 2. Uncoated macroreticular resin after contact with blood.
Fig. 3. Albumin-coated macroreticular resin after contact with blood.

dehyde (GA) in PBS for 1 h. The traces of GA were inactivated by incubation in a solution of lysine in PBS for 1 h and by a final wash with PBS. The resin was then washed with saline until the affluent showed no traces of phosphate and cold-stored in saline. The coated resin was sterilized by γ-radiation: 2.5 *M* rad were used.

The surface morphology of the particles was examined with a JSM-U3 scanning electron microscope. For blood-particle interaction tests, the particles were preequlibrated in PBS + ACD solution. Fresh human blood containing ACD was then added to the particles. The blood was removed after 30 min and the particles were thoroughly washed with PBS + ACD. After fixation with glutaradeldehyde and osmium tetraoxide, the particles were dehydrated, critical point dried and vacuum coated with gold paladium.

The surface of an uncoated macroreticular resin, after 30 min contact with blood, is shown in figure 2. Adsorbed proteins and thrombocytes are quite evident. In contrast with the uncoated resin, the properly coated resin surface shown in figure 3 is smooth and clean of settled blood particles.

Bilirubin Removal by Hemoperfusion

In vivo studies of the removal of bilirubin from the blood by HP requires a suitable jaundiced animal model. Two such models, both utilizing dogs, are considered here.

Hyperbilirubinemia by a Choledocho-Suprarenal Vein Shunt

Mongrel dogs 15–30 kg were anesthetized by intravenous sodium pentobarbital (25–30 mg/kg b.w.). The common bile duct was divided, the distal end ligated and a 2-mm catheter was introduced into the proximal duct lumen. A separate catheter was introduced into the inferior vena cava through a right suprarenal vein. The catheters were brought out by separate incisions and connected via a 3-way stopcock. Thus, the bile could flow freely into the vena cava or to drain into a collecting bag. By closing the tap, a simple obstructive jaundice could also be obtained. The choledocho-suprarenal vein shunt yielded 20–50 mg% total bilirubin concentrations for relatively long periods, as well as some days of increased unconjugated bilirubin (1–4 mg%) levels. The latter were determined by the *Weber and Schalm* [36] extraction method.

The anesthetized dogs were intubated and connected to the HP column via the femoral artery and vein. The 'shunted' dogs were given 250 IU/kg b.w. heparin intravenously and subsequent doses of 100 IU/kg b.w. every hour. The Plexiglass column contained 200 ml macroreticular albumin-coated resin particles which were preequilibrated by recirculating 200 ml heparinized saline (10 IU/ml) for 1 h. The hematological, chemical and hemodynamic data are given elsewhere [37]. Here, we relate only to the bilirubin removal characteristics.

The results of the HP carried on 3 dogs are presented in figure 4. It is noteworthy that the in vivo and the in vitro HP experiments were carried out with a resin to blood volume ratio of 0.1–0.2, and with a flow rate corresponding to the total blood volume passing the column in 10–20 min. Inspection of figures 1 and 4 shows that the percent bilirubin retained in the blood of the dogs after HP is higher than in the in vitro experiments. This is probably due to the continuous equilibration of the bilirubin between the plasma and the extravascular bilirubin pools which takes place during the HP. The latter is demonstrated in figure 4 by comparison with data obtained from exchange transfusion (ET) of jaundiced babies. Although the comparison of babies to dogs is inappropriate, figure 4 serves to demonstrate the bilirubin rebound after the ET and the apparent lack of it in these HP experiments. Since the unconjugated bilirubin represents only some 10% of the total bilirubin concentration, the decrease in total bilirubin concentration during HP indicates good adsorption of the conjugated bilirubin. However, the data indicate [33] the preferential adsorption of the unconjugated bilirubin.

Hyperbilirubinemia by Bilirubin Infusion

To obtain higher levels of unconjugated bilirubin, a bilirubin infusion procedure was utilized on healthy dogs. A sterile bilirubin solution of 5 mg/ml in 0.1 *N* Na_2CO_3 was infused at a rate approximated by estimating the natural bilirubin clearance of the dog.

Figure 5 represents an experiment with a bilirubin infusion rate of 0.15 ml/min/kg b.w. for 15 min followed by 0.05 ml/min/kg b.w. Obviously, the infu-

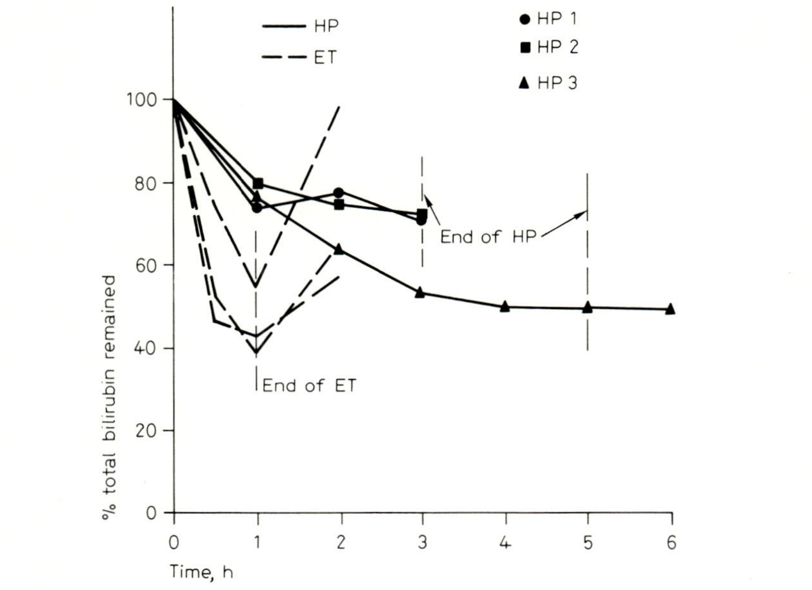

4

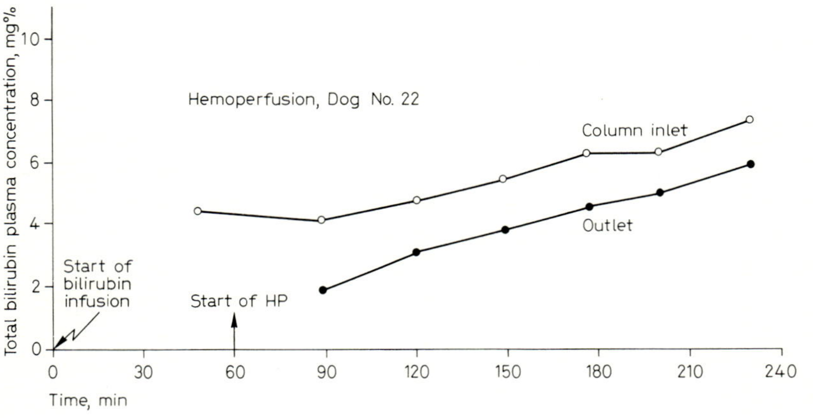

5

Fig. 4. Percent of the initial total bilirubin concentration which remains in blood during hemoperfusion of dogs. Comparison with exchange transfusion data on 3 newborn babies. Column volume 200 ml. Blood flow rate 260, 206 and 150 ml/min for HP. No. 1, 2 and 3, respectively.

Fig. 5. Inlet and outlet bilirubin concentration during hemoperfusion with bilirubin infusion of healthy dog. 0.15 ml/min/kg b.w. of 5 mg/ml bilirubin in 0.1 *M* Na_2CO_3 were infused for 15 min followed by 0.05 ml/min/kg b.w.

sion rate exceeded the natural clearance of bilirubin. It is also evident that the bilirubin clearance by the 80 ml macroreticular resin column (3–8 ml/min) was insufficient to change the particular slope of the bilirubin curve. However, the amount of bilirubin removed is rather large: the clearance data show that 41 mg of bilirubin was removed on the 80-ml resin column during 3 h. Relating these results to a human newborn baby with, say, 200 ml blood and a mean bilirubin concentration of 5 mg%, indicates that a column with 40 ml resin can remove some 20 mg bilirubin in 3 h. In other words the column can remove in 3 h four times the amount of bilirubin initially present in the blood (assuming a hematocrit of 50%).

The Heparinization Procedure

Proper heparinization is required to prevent clotting or bleeding during, or after, the extracorporeal procedure.

Gotch and Keen's [34] model was adopted here for the heparinization of 8–14 kg female Baboon monkeys. In the heparin level of 60–180 IU/kg b.w. used here, the protrombin time (PT) was found to be a suitable correlation parameter. Constant level of heparinization is achieved by injection of an initial heparin bolus and then infusing heparin so as to overcome the natural decay.

In vivo Hemoperfusion of Baboons

Having established the individual heparinization required to maintain the different baboons at a desired 'response' level, the animals were first put through 'control' runs which simulated the HP procedure without actually performing the perfusion through the column. These 'control' experiments served to verify the reliability of the a priori predicted heparinization procedure as well as provide a reference for comparing the subsequent resin HP runs. Hematological and coagulation data were taken before, during and after the experiments. The preliminary data for Baboon No. 4 are presented in table I. Note that a constant level of heparinization was achieved. The changes in thrombocytes, fibrinogen level and in platelet aggregation in the HP run were not significantly different from those obtained in the control experiment. Platelet aggregation is affected by the heparin level and drops to a normal value a day after the HP. As noted by the data for the column inlet and outlet, the resin column does not seem to affect the parameters tested.

The hemodynamics of the baboons were constant during the 'control' experiments. ECG was continuously monitored. The heart rate in the control experiment of baboon No. 4 was 90–120 beats/min; respiration movements

Table I. Hematological and coagulation data: comparision of effects of HP with those of controlled heparinization only

Test	System	0 min	100 min		180 min	
			in	out	in	out
Platelets $\times 10^{-5}$ µl	HP	3.1	2.98	2.8	2.66	2.60
	control	2.2	2.15		2.3	
Platelet aggregation	HP	**	***	***	***	***
	control	*	***		****	
Fibrinogen, mg %	HP	290	237	228	230	230
	control	240	173		185	
Ca^{++}, mg %	HP	7.7	8.8	9	10	9.8
	control	9.3	9.2		9	
PT, s	HP	15	17	17	17.1	17.5
	control	14	21.7		20.5	
APTT, s	HP	25.1	37	37.5	36	36.4
	control	25	46		46.5	

* normal, <30 s; ** 30–40 s; *** 40–60 s; **** >60 s.

14–16/min, blood pressure average 105–115 mm Hg. The only effect noticed on the ECG was the inversion of the T wave during deep anesthesia by Nembutal. At the end of the experiment, the ECG came back to normal. During the HP the heart rate variations were 108–130 beats/min; blood pressure: 120/70–150/65 mm Hg; respiration: 17–23 breaths/min. The blood gases ranged in the normal level pCO_2: 43–47; pO_2: 75–75; pH: 7.38–7.31. The animal was not assisted. The HP were carried out safely without impairing the well-being of the animals and the baboons withstood repeated HPs without any ill effects.

Finally, it is noteworthy that whereas a fraction of the tested hormones (T_4, cortisol and aldosterone) is adsorbed by the macroreticular resin in vitro, this adsorption is insignificant when occurring in vivo. Evidently the production rate of the hormones, probably enhanced by a stress signal, highly exceeds their elimination rate by the column.

Conclusions

The macroreticular anion exchange resin selected here was found to remove unconjugated bilirubin even from blood containing high concentrations of conjugated bilirubin. Proper coating with a thin layer of albumin assures biocompatibility. Changes in thrombocytes, fibrinogen, and platelet aggregation in the HP run were not different from those realised in the control experiment.

The amount of bilirubin removed from the blood during HP of dogs 'jaundiced' by either choledocho-suprarenal vein shunting or direct infusion of bilirubin assures the efficient application of this small column (containing ~10% of the total blood volume) to jaundiced babies.

Preliminary safety tests with baboons established a reasonable procedure for continuous heparinization. Furthermore, the hematological data indicated that the coagulation factors were not affected by the resin HP.

The experimental results encourage the anticipated application of the resin column to the clinical treatment of babies with unconjugated hyperbilirubinemia.

Acknowledgement

The initial steps of this research program were supported by the Israel National Council for Research and development and the GSF München, FRG. Most of the work reported here was supported by the MEP Fund of the Women's Division, American Technion Society, USA. Our sincere gratitude is given for this trust and support.

Summary

The application of an anionic macroreticular ion exchange resin, coated with a thin cross-linked albumin layer, as a hemoperfusion device for the removal of unconjugated bilirubin from the blood of hyperbilirubinemic newborn babies is reviewed. In vivo hemoperfusion runs with hyperbilirubinemic animal models – either by a choledocho-suprarenal vein shunt or by direct infusion of bilirubin into the vein – showed that a 40-ml resin column can remove some 20 mg bilirubin in 3 h. Hemoperfusion of female 8–14 kg baboons showed no significant effect of the column on blood chemistry and coagulation factors and repeated runs had no ill effects.

References

1 Chang, T.M.S.: Semipermeable aqueous microcapsules (artificial cells) with emphasis on experiments in an extracorporeal shunt system. Trans. Am. Soc. artif. internal Organs *12:* 13 (1966).

2 Yatzidis, H.: A convenient hemoperfusion microapparatus over charcoal for the treatment of endogenous and exogenous intoxications. Its use as an artificial kidney. Proc. Eur. Dial. Transplant Ass. *1:* 83 (1964).

3 Muirhead, E.E.; Reid, A.F.: A resin artificial kidney. J. Lab. clin. Med. *33:* 841–844 (1948).

4 Bronniman, P.; Pini, S.: Construction of an artificial kidney based on the physicochemical properties of the exchange resins. Trans. Am. Soc. artif. internal Organs *1:* 16 (1955).

5 Rosenbaum, J.L.; Kramer, M.S.; Raja, R.; Boreyko, C.: Resin hemoperfusion: A new treatment for acute drug intoxication. New Engl. J. Med. *184:* 874 (1971).

6 Rosenbaum, J.: Amberlite hemoperfusion in detoxification; in Proc. The S. Neaman Workshop on Hemoperfusion, Haifa 1979, pp. 105–107.

7 Klinkmann, H.; Falkenhagen, D.; Courtney, J.M.: Blood purification by hemoperfusion. Int. J. artif. Organs *2:* 296–308 (1979).

8 Martensson, E.; Selander, D.; Wickstrom, I.; Ahlmen, J.: Hemoperfusion with amberlite resin in the treatment of self-poisoning. Acta med. scand. *207:* 455–460 (1980).

9 Sideman, S.; Manas-Zloczower, I.: Topic in hemoperfusion: Classification of published work, in Sideman, Chang, Hemoperfusion: Kidney and liver supports and detoxification, part 1, pp. 409–468 (Hemisphere-McGraw Hill, New York 1980).

10 Sideman, S.; Manas-Zloczower, I.: Topic in hemoperfusion: Classification of published work – update; in Sideman, Chang, Hemoperfusion: Kidney and liver supports and detoxification, part II, Proc. The Neaman Workshop, Haifa (Hemisphere-McGraw-Hill, New York 1980).

11 Sideman, S.; Chang, T.M.S.: Hemoperfusion: Kidney and liver support and detoxification, part 1. Proc. Int. Symp. Technion, Haifa 1979 (Hemisphere-McGraw-Hill, New York 1980).

12 Sideman, S.; Chang, T.M.S.: Hemoperfusion: Kidney and liver support and detoxification, part II. Proc. S. Neaman Workshop, Beit Oren, Haifa 1979 (S. Neaman Institute for Advanced Studies on Science and Technology, 1980).

13 Sideman, S.; Chang, T.M.S.: Summary and Abstracts of the International Symposium on Hemoperfusion: Kidney and liver supports and detoxification, Aug. 15–16 Haifa, Israel. Artif. Organs *3:* 393–402 (1979).

14 Sideman, S.; Chang, T.M.S.: Hemoperfusion – State-of-the-art and future requirements. Artif. Organs *4:* 70–75 (1980).

15 Berk, P.D.: A computer simulation study relating to the treatment of fulminant hepatic failure by hemoperfusion. Proc. Soc. exp. Biol. Med. *155:* 535 (1977).

16 Lie, T.S.; Kim, W.I.; Holst, A.; Grunn, U.; Rommelsheim, K.: Treatment of extrahepatic occlusive jaundice with activated charcoal hemoperfusion in dogs. Acta hepato-gastro-enter. *23:* 262 (1976).

17 Dunlop, E.H.; Jughes, R.D.; Williams, R.: Physicochemical aspects of the removal of protein bound substances by charcoal and other adsorbents of potential value in systems of artificial liver support. II. Kinetics of removal. Bio-Eng. Comput. *16:* 350–362 (1978).

18 Willson, R.A.; Hofmann, A.F.; Kuster, G.G.R.: Toward and artificial liver. II. Removal of cholephillic anions from dogs with biliary obstruction by hemoperfusion through charged and uncharged resins. Gastroenterology *66:* 95 (1974).

19 Lopukhin, U.M.; Shurkalin, B.K.; Leykin, U.A.; Evseev, N.G.; Molodenkov, M.N.; Kuznetzov, V.N.; Gorchakov, V.D.; Blagosklonov, A.S.: Bilirubin removal by anion-exchange resin. Lancet *ii:* 461 (1975).

20 Lopukhin, U.M.; Molodenkov, M.N.; Leykin, U.A.; Gorchakov, V.D.; Evseev, N.G.; Ryabov, A.V.: Removal of plasma bilirubin by hemoperfusion in dogs. Am. J. Gastroenterol. *68:* 345 (1977).

21 Hughes, R.D.; Ton, H.Y.; Langley, P.G.; Williams, R.: The use of an in vitro haemoperfusion circuit to evaluate the blood compatibility of albumin-coated Amberlite XAD-7 resin. Int. J. artif. Organs *1:* 129 (1978).

22 Hughes, R.; Ton, H.Y.; Langley, P.; Davies, M.; Hanid, M.A.; Mellon, P.; Silk, D.B.A.; Williams, R.: Albumin-coated Amberlite XAD-7 resin for hemoperfusion in acute liver failure. II. In vivo evaluation. Artif. Organs *3:* 23 (1979).

23 Scharschmidt, B.F.; Martin, J.F.; Shapiro, L.J.; Plotz, P.H.; Berk, P.D.: Hemoperfusion through albumin-conjugated agarose gel for the treatment of neonatal jaundice in premature rhesus monkeys. J. Lab. clin. Med. *89:* 101 (1977).

24 Sideman, S.; Mor, L.; Rousseau, I.; Brandes, J.M.; Ben-Arie, D.: Removal of bilirubin from the blood of jaundiced infants; in Kenedi, Courtney, Gaylor, Gilchrist: Artificial Organs, Proc. 2nd Strathclyde Bioengineering Seminar, 1976, pp. 413–424 (Maxmillan, London 1977).

25 Sideman, S.; Mor, L.; Brandes, J.M.: Removal of bilirubin by hemoperfusion with ion exchangers. (Abstract) Am. Soc. artif. internal Organs *8:* 62 (1979): Trans Am. Soc. artif. internal Organs *25:* 497–501 (1979).

26 Sideman, S.; Mor, L.; Fishler, L.S.; Thaler, I.; Brandes, J.M.: Bilirubin removal by sorbent hemoperfusion from jaundiced blood; in Artificial liver: Proc. Int. Symp. Artificial Liver Support, Celle 1980 (Springer, Berlin, in press).

27 Sideman, S.; Mor, L.; Brandes, J.M.: Sorption of bilirubin by anion exchange resins in vitro. Am. Soc. artif. internal Organs J. *3:* 85 (1980).

28 Saveliera, G.M.; Segienko, N.S.; Leikin, J.A.: Using of Ionex exchanging resins for removal of indirect bilirubin in hemolysing disease of newborn. Artif. Organs *4:* 148 (1980).

29 Ton, H.Y.; Hughes, R.D.; Silk, D.B.A.; Williams, R.: Albumin-coated Amberlite XAD-7 resin for hemoperfusion in acute liver failure. I. Adsorption studies. Artif. Organs *3:* 20 (1979).

30 Chang, T.M.S.: Removal of endogenous and exogenous toxins by a microencapsulated absorbent. Can. J. Physiol. Pharmacol. *47:* 1043–1045 (1969).

31 Sideman, S.; Hoffer, E.; Mor, L.; Brandes, J.M.; Rousseau, I.; Better, O.; Ben-Arie, D.; Lupovitch, S.: Biocompatibility studies of hemoperfusion systems for liver and kidney support; in Chang, Artificial liver and artificial cells, pp. 173–182 (Plenum Press, New York 1978).

32 Koshino, I.; Matsushita, M.; Kawamata, T.; Kondo, M.; Nakajima, Y.; Kon, T.; Kasai, T.: Improvement of XAD-4 Resin by various coating (Abstract). Am. Soc. artif. internal Organs *8:* 61 (1979).

33 Shapiro, W.B.; Faubert, P.F.; Chou, S.Y.; Porush, J.G.: Low dose heparin in the high risk bleeding hemodialysis patient monitored by activated partial thromboplastin time. Dial. Transplant. *9:* 322 (1980).

34 Gotch, F.A.; Keen, M.L.: Precise control of minimal heparinization for high bleeding risk hemodialysis. Trans. Am. Soc. artif. internal Organs *23:* 168 (1977).

35 Sideman, S.; Mor, L.; Brandes, J.M.; Lupovitch, S.: Preparation of a biocompatible albumin-coated ion exchange resin for bilirubin removal from the blood of jaundiced newborn. Technion R&D Report No. 80 to Israel Nat. Council for R&D and GSF, Munchen 1980 (Submitted for publication).

36 Weber, A.P.; Schalm, L.: Quantitative separation and determination of bilirubin in human serum. Clinica chim. Acta *7:* 805 (1962).

37 Mor, L.; Thaler, I.; Brandes, J.M.; Sideman, S.: In vito hemoperfusion studies for bilirubin removal from jaundiced dogs. Int. I. artif. Organs *4:* (1981).

S. Sideman, MD, Department of Chemical Engineering, Technion,
Israel Institute of Technology, Haifa 32000 (Israel)

Contr. Nephrol., vol. 29, pp. 101–113 (Karger, Basel 1982)

Hemoperfusion in Toxic Ingestions and Hepatic Encephalopathy: Have the Expectations Been Achieved?

M.C. Gelfand

Georgetown University Medical Center, Washington, D.C., USA

Although sorbents, especially charcoal, were known as a medicinal adjunct in ancient Greece and China, it is *Muirhead and Reid* [1] who receive credit for having introduced the idea of hemoperfusion into clinical medicine in 1948. These authors demonstrated in vitro that certain sorbents have the capacity to remove toxins directly from blood. 10 years later, *Schreiner* [2] provided the classical demonstration of the capacity of an ion-exchange resin column to treat a patient with pentobarbital poisoning. From these pioneering studies, a number of investigations into the clinical use of sorbents led to the currently available devices used for the treatment of drug intoxication throughout the world. These devices also have applicability in the treatment of other syndromes associated with the accumulation of toxins in the circulation including the coma of hepatic failure and renal failure. The development of the clinical applicability of hemoperfusion was delayed because of the demonstration that the procedure as performed by *Schreiner* [2] was associated with significant potential complications including pyrogenic reactions, electrolyte disturbances, and hemolysis of blood passing over the column [3, 4]. The quest was, therefore, initiated to find a more biocompatible substance which could act as a sorbent in this newly defined system.

In 1964, *Yatzidis* [5] demonstrated that a column containing 200 g of activated charcoal particles could adsorb from plasma 1–2 g of short- and long-acting barbiturates as well as salicylic acid and glutethimide. *Yatzidis* et al. [6] used these findings in support of a clinical trial in 1965 where 2 patients with barbiturate poisoning were treated by charcoal hemoperfusion. Both patients recovered consciousness after three to five hemoperfusions of 1 h each. The side effects of this charcoal hemoperfusion procedure were minimal except for depletion of platelets and reduction in clotting factors. The work of *Yatzidis* brought significant interest in the development of sorbent hemoperfusion. However, it became apparent in subsequent animal studies that in fact charcoal hemoperfusion might be associated with more significant complications than

Table I. Removal[a] of poisons by hemoperfusion

Drug or substance	coated for uncoated charcoal hemoperfusion			XAD-2 or XAD-4 resin hemoperfusion		
	plasma extraction ratio	clearance	mg or (%) drug removed	plasma extraction ratio	clearance	mg or (%) drug removed
Acetaminophen	0.5	90	(13)	0.7	140	NA
Amobarbital	0.5	120	(19)	0.9	260	1,200 (15)
Carbromal	0.6	250	NA	1.0	300	NA
Digoxin	0.3	85	0.5 (5)	0.5	110	0.05 (3)
Ethchlorvynol	0.7	173	(30?)	1.0	200	2,000 (35)
Glutethimide	0.7	200	(6)	0.8	170	3,000
Paraquat	0.6	65	220 (2)	0.9	NA	NA
Phenobarbital	0.5	130	1,500 (10)	0.9	280	220 (2)
Salicylates	0.5	120	5,000 (50?)	–	–	–
Theophylline	0.7	85[b]	NA	0.8	185	NA
Tricyclics	0.4	100	NA	0.8	185	260 (7)

NA = Not available
[a] = Calculated at similar conditions of blood flow (Q_B = 200–300 ml/min) from world literature.
[b] Q_B = 90 ml/min.

originally found. These complications included significant platelet loss and the possibility of embolization of particles of charcoal from the hemoperfusion device.

Subsequent efforts to develop safe, effective sorbent hemoperfusion systems, therefore, followed four major lines. In the first line, *Rosenbaum* et al. [7] continued to pursue the use of an ion-exchange sorbent. This line, although showing some promise with the IR 100 H cartridge, did not produce a system safe enough for human clinical use. The second line pursued by *Rosenbaum* et al. [7] involved the use of a nonionic microporous resin such as the XAD-2 and XAD-4 materials. These polystyrenes amberlite series sorbents were demonstrated to be extremely effective in the removal of a variety of poisons (table I) and represent devices which are commercially available and in wide use today.

Chang et al. [8] followed up on *Yatzidis's* work continuing to use charcoal as the basic sorbent but ingeniously encapsulating the charcoal particles in albumin or albumin-collodion to enhance its biocompatibility and to prevent possibility of embolization of the charcoal material. *Chang's* [9] highly important work demonstrated the applicability of this ACAC charcoal hemoperfusion system not only in the treatment of toxic ingestions but also in the treatment of hepatic coma and uremia. In subsequent developments, charcoal was successfully encapsulated in acrylic hydrogel materials, again, with the purpose of enhancing biocompatibility and preventing embolization of charcoal. These encapsulated charcoal systems have evolved into the Smith and Nephew Hemacol device [10], the Gambro Hemoadsorba device and other commercial systems. *Hill* et al. [11] ingeniously designed an uncoated device in which the granular charcoal was fixed to a polyethylene backing and wound into a spiral. This device, known as the Hemodetoxifier produced by Becton-Dickinson, USA, remains the only commercially available uncoated charcoal sorbent device.

With the rebirth of the use of sorbents in modern medicine as a clinical treatment of toxic ingestion as the results of work of *Schreiner, Rosenbaum, Chang,* and others over the last 25 years, it is not inappropriate to pose the question that will be the crux of this paper: Have the expectations for hemoperfusion in acute poisoning been achieved? The expectations in the treatment of acute poisoning which sorbent hemoperfusion should achieve include safety, efficiency, and effectiveness. In regard to safety the system must be nontoxic, per se, should not result in sorbent embolization, and should have reasonably satisfactory biocompatibility. As far as efficiency is concerned, the device should be easy to use and should have a low cost/benefit ratio. At the very least, it should be the best available therapy. As far as effectiveness is concerned, there must be demonstrable drug removal, a reduced morbidity, and an increased survival. In the remainder of this paper we will examine whether or not sorbent hemoperfusion has achieved these goals as it is used in the treatment of toxin ingestions or the coma associated with hepatic encephalopathy.

Safety

We have already commented above on the safety of commercially available hemoperfusion devices. In general, these devices are now compatible within the guidelines set for safety of intravenous fluids and devices coming in contact with circulation. *Fennimore* et al. [10] demonstrated with the Smith and Nephew acrylic hydrogel-coated column that the affluent contains an amount of particulate material which is acceptable under the guidelines established by the British standard for infusion fluids. Other columns have been similarly demonstrated to have no significant release of particulate material.

Perhaps the major continuing problem with some hemoperfusion devices is the loss of platelets as a result of this procedure. Although a reasonably biocompatible material, some of the coated or uncoated sorbents currently in use are nevertheless inherently destructive of platelets which soon thereafter are removed from the circulation. An additional thrombocytopenic factor might be the development of aggregates of platelets within the circulation perhaps as a result of the release of platelet aggregating factors on contact with some sorbents [12]. For the most part, in the treatment of toxic ingestions, thrombocytopenia does not become a significant problem. This is because in the vast majority of instances patients are reasonably healthy at the onset of the procedure and only one to three procedures are usually required. In most cases, therefore, platelet levels return to normal in a short period of time. As we will see below, however, in cases of hepatic failure where thrombocytopenia exists even before hemoperfusion, platelet depletion resulting from less blood-compatible devices can be seriously exacerbated in most cases requiring replacement of platelets to maintain adequate platelet levels. Hemolysis of red cells, although potentially a problem, does not appear to be a significant problem as the result of hemoperfusion, especially in short-term situations such as the treatment of drug intoxications [13].

Efficiency

Currently available hemoperfusion systems have been developed to provide a system which is easy to use and of relatively low cost. The first point has not in fact been debated since, in general, hemoperfusion systems are easier to use than hemodialysis in most cases. The second statement, however, that hemoperfusion represents a relatively low-cost procedure has been debated. At a cost of approximately $ 300 per treatment, the procedure is roughly comparable to a single acute hemodialysis procedure in hospitals in the United States. In the same hospitals, a single day's stay in an Intensive Care Unit costs more than the costs of a hemoperfusion treatment. If hemoperfusion in drug intoxication is capable of reducing the Intensive Care hospital stay of the patient by 1 day, it at least covers the costs of the treatment in the money saved by reducing the duration of the hospital stay. This point has been questioned by *Bismuth* et al. [14], who stated that in the French hospital system, the cost of hemoperfusion appeared to outweigh the potential benefit of the therapy. Nevertheless animal toxicological and clinical studies strongly suggest that coma time is significantly reduced by hemoperfusion potentially providing the opportunity for earlier discharge of the patient. Of course, if hemoperfusion in the treatment of toxic ingestions can be demonstrated to in fact provide the best *available* therapy (even if not the best potentially available therapy) then the issue of cost/benefit ratio is of considerably less significance. It is clear that in most instances of serious toxic ingestions, hemoperfusion does in fact provide the best available therapy. Comparing hemoperfusion to other facilitated drug removal treatments, for example, peritoneal or hemodialysis, reveals that hemoperfusion is two- to tenfold superior in the removal of toxins. Moreover, in animal studies comparing hemoperfusion to peritoneal or hemodialysis in experimental barbiturate intoxication, dogs recovered significantly faster from coma if treated with hemoperfusion compared to other modalities [15].

Effectiveness

In evaluating whether or not hemoperfusion has achieved the expectations of its proponents, the evaluation of the effectiveness of hemoperfusion must be considered the paramount consideration (providing that the procedure passes toxicity testing). In view of the fact that devices have been developed which are relatively nontoxic and reasonably biocompatible, the major concern then becomes one of effectiveness.

Drug Removal

To be considered an effective device, the sorbent system must be demonstrated to be capable of removing drugs from the circulation. As shown in table I, charcoal and resin sorbent systems have clearly demonstrated a capacity to remove significant amounts of various drugs. In most cases, the XAD-4 resin system appears to be somewhat superior to charcoal systems but both are, in general, highly efficient in removing drugs. This is not to stay that drug removal can be accomplished under all conditions. *Farrell* [16] has outlined a number of factors which, if present, inhibit the success of hemoperfusion in the treatment of acute poisoning (table II). While we certainly agree that it is unlikely that hemoperfusion will be of any benefit in counteracting toxic ingestions associated with drugs with very rapid action such as cyanide or in drugs with metabolic elimination rates exceeding hemoperfusion removal rates, it is not clear that Farrell's points for 5, 6, and 7 are in fact completely valid. Paraquat intoxication, for

Table II. Factors mitigating against use of hemoperfusion in acute poisoning [modified from ref. 16]

(1)	Drug with rapid action (e.g. cyanides)
(2)	Drug with metabolic elimination rates exceeding hemoperfusion removal rates
(3)	Drugs removal by dialysis which produce concomitant acidosis (e.g. ASA)
(4)	Drug with irreversible effects (e.g. paraquat?)
(5)	Drug with large volume of distribution (e.g. tricyclics?)
(6)	Drug without serious toxic effects (e.g. valium?)
(7)	Drug with effective antagonists (e.g. paracetamol/cysteamine?)

example, which is felt to have irreversible effects, has apparently been successfully treated with hemoperfusion whereas it is virtually universally fatal when untreated. Patients who ingested drugs such as tricyclics may, in fact, have benefitted from hemoperfusion in spite of the fact that these agents distribute in very large total body volumes. Moreover, there is the question whether in fact there are many (if any) drugs without serious toxic effects. Overdosage with Valium has in fact been associated with serious complications. In such cases, hemoperfusion may in fact be of significant benefit.

A special case wherein other forms of facilitated drug removal such as hemodialysis or peritoneal dialysis may have specific benefit is the situation where the drug involved in the toxic ingestion is associated with concomitant metabolic acidosis such as with salicylic acid. In such a case, hemodialysis may be superior since it is capable of treating the concomitant acidosis simultaneously.

In considering the circumstances which present the appropriate clinical situation favoring remcval of various drugs of hemoperfusion, it is reasonable to consider the critical factors which affect drug removal by hemoperfusion. Firstly, various drugs have various capacities to be bound by the sorbent. A listing of potentially hemoadsorbable drugs and toxins has been reported previously [13]. Assuming the potential adsorbability of the drug, one then needs to be aware of the volume of tissue distribution and the intercompartmental rate. *Gibson* [17], *Farrell* [16], and others have pointed out that drugs with particularly large volumes of distribution or distribution within tissue spaces not available to removal from the central compartment inhibit the effectiveness of hemoperfusion. In addition, of paramount importance is the facility with which a drug can transfer from its storage compartment to the central compartment (circulating blood volume) for removal by the sorbent. In the case of glutethimide, for example, the drug is largely distributed within adipose tissues of the body. For hemoperfusion to be effective, it might have to be repeated two or three times thereby allowing

Table III. The controversy hemoperfusion for acute poisoning

Pro (International Workshop on Hemoperfusion, Haifa, Israel 1979)
Hemoperfusion is indicated for serious toxic ingestion in the presence of:

(1) Hypoventilation, hypothermia, hypotension, non-responsiveness despite supportive measures
(2) Lethal blood concentration of one or more potentially adsorbable drugs
(3) Prolonged coma associated with pneumonia or severe COPD

Con

(1) Conservative medical management works [21]
(2) Mortality rates are low in poisoning [22]
(3) Complications of hemoperfusion are not insignificant [14]

the relatively slow movement of drug from adipose tissue into the central compartment for removal. Concerning tricyclics wherein there is a large volume of distribution, i.e., little drug is actually present in the circulating central compartment, the issue remains unresolved as to whether hemoperfusion is of any benefit at all.

Under appropriate conditions, therefore, there is little doubt that hemoperfusion is effective in removing a variety of toxins directly from the blood. We next ask whether hemoperfusion has been shown to be of benefit in either reducing morbidity (i.e., reducing coma time) or enhancing survival. Unfortunately, the data to answer these questions are scant or in fact unavailable. In vivo animal studies have demonstrated the superiority of hemoperfusion to hemodialysis or no treatment in reducing the duration of coma in barbiturate-intoxicated dogs [15]. For obvious reasons, such studies have not been done in humans and it is unlikely that they will ever be done in a controlled fashion.

As far as enhancing survival time, the controversy continues to rage as to whether hemoperfusion does in fact save lives. Proponents of hemoperfusion for the treatment of acute intoxications line up behind the position put forward by members of the International Workshop on Hemoperfusion held in Haifa, Israel, in 1979 (table III). These proponents contend that if hemoperfusion is used in instances where there is clearly a serious intoxication with a reasonably high probability of mortality, it is indicated and it is likely to be of benefit. This position is supported by a number of uncontrolled studies demonstrating a clearly satisfactory result using hemoperfusion in cases of serious intoxication. In addition, in a retrospective study by *Hampel* et al. [18] controlling for the seriousness of intoxication in 52 untreated patients with grade III or IV coma due to hypnotic ingestion, there were 10 deaths. In contrast, of 14 patients receiving hemoperfusion under similar circumstances there was only one death.

In contrast, detractors point to the issues shown in table III. They assert that conservative medical management is as effective as hemoperfusion since mortality rates are so very low anyway and since complications which might arise from hemoperfusion are not in fact insignificant. This issue remains acute and unresolved; however, opinion appears to favor the position posed by the International Hemoperfusion Workshop Group.

Summary

In summary, the expectations of the fathers of clinical hemoperfusion (table IV) have generally been achieved. Safe and efficient devices are available commercially to allow hemoperfusion in cases of toxic ingestions by most reasonably staffed hospitals throughout the world. With respect to effectiveness, only the clear capacity of hemoperfusion systems to effect drug removal has been demonstrated. The capacity of hemoperfusion in acute poisoning either to reduce morbidity or increase survival have not been demonstrated conclusively by any controlled human study of which I am aware. Nevertheless, the preponderance of evidence strongly supports the position of the International Workshop on Hemoperfusion of 1979. Further controlled trials are, however, highly desirable and needed as are controlled investigations into the possibility that hemoperfusion may have a beneficial effect in potentially preventing long-term toxic effects of various poisonings.

Hemoperfusion in Hepatic Failure

Although the expectations of the early proponents of hemoperfusion in the treatment of hepatic coma were considerably more restrained than those of early proponents of hemoperfusion in acute ingestions, even these modest expectations have been only partially achieved by clinical results to date.

The expectations for hemoperfusion in hepatic coma are outlined in table V. The safety-related issues of biocompatibility, nontoxicity, per se, and absence of possible embolization have basically been covered in the appropriate sections concerning hemoperfusion in toxic ingestions. Of special interest in the area of hemoperfusion in hepatic coma, however, is the additional complication that patients with hepatic failure tend to arrive for treatment with already established thrombocytopenia and deficiencies in circulating clotting factors. To overcome these problems, we have recommended the infusion of fresh frozen plasma (1 unit per 10 kg body weight) and platelets (1 unit for 10 kg body weight) at the end of each hemoperfusion procedure for patients with hepatic coma [19]. Other systems which would be more biocompatible are under investigation at this time.

Table IV. Expectations for hemoperfusion in acute poisoning

Safety	
Nontoxic, per se	achieved
No embolization	achieved
Biocompatibility	partly achieved
Efficiency	
Ease of use	achieved
Low cost/benefit ratio	achieved
Best available therapy	achieved
Efficacy	
Drug removal	achieved
Reduced morbidity	no controlled trials
Increased survival	no controlled trials
Preventive benefit	under investigation

Table V. Expectations for hemoperfusion in hepatic coma

Safety
Biocompatible/nontoxic per se
No embolization
Does not remove necessary circulating substances
Efficacy
Remove toxins
Reverse coma
Increase survival
Best available therapy

Effectiveness of Hemoperfusion in Hepatic Coma

As far as efficacy of hemoperfusion in coma is concerned, clinical reports over the last 20 years since *Chang* first attempted to treat hepatic encephalopathy with the ACAC device and then the King's College group reported the first apparently successful clinical trial [20] have been quite variable. Indeed, the same British group has reported both very positive results and relatively negative results, within a short period of time. Nevertheless, it is reasonably clear that hemoperfusion is potentially capable of removing a variety of toxins which have been implicated in the pathogenesis of hepatic coma (table VI).

Although it remains unclear as to which toxin or toxins are in fact responsible for the coma associated with hepatic failure, the toxins that are listed are able to cause coma in appropriate doses when infused into laboratory animals. Moreover, these agents are found in abnormal concentrations in patients with he-

Table VI. Effect of hemoperfusion in toxins implicated in the pathogenesis of hepatic coma

Toxin	Abnormality	Effect of hemoperfusion
Ammonia	increased [23]	decreases [31]
False neurotransmitters (e.g. octopamine)	increased [24]	decreases [32]
Free fatty acids	increased [25]	decreases [33]
Phenols	increased [26]	decreases [34]
Mercaptans	increased [27]	decreases [35]
Aromatic amino acids	increased [28]	decreases [31]
Ratio of branched to aromatic amino acids	decreased [29]	increases [30]
CSF cyclic AMP	decreased [30]	increases [30]

Table VII. Expectations for hemoperfusion in hepatic coma

Safety	
Biocompatible/nontoxic per se	partially achieved
No embolization	partially achieved
Does not remove necessary circulating substance	not achieved
Efficacy	
Removes toxins	partially achieved
Reverses coma	no controlled trails
Increases survival	no controlled trails
Best available therapy	no controlled trails
Preventive therapy	under investigation

patic coma. This situation is not terribly dissimilar from the uremic syndrome. The uremic toxin(s) remains just as elusive in 1981 as it was 100 years ago, however, hemodialysis and peritoneal dialysis are known effectively to remove whatever the uremic toxin(s) might in fact be.

While it would not be disputed by us that the ultimate criterion by which to measure the efficacy of hemoperfusion in hepatic coma should be patient survival, it is, nevertheless, clear that the reversal of coma for a more or less sustained period of time presents another standard by which efficacy could be assessed. Just as in chronic renal failure where hemodialysis certainly does not reverse the underlying pathology, hemoperfusion in hepatic coma while not reversing the hepatic failure may in fact reduce or reverse coma. Moreover, as in acute renal failure, the maintenance of consciousness might allow time for the regeneration of adequate hepatic tissue to sustain life. As shown in table VII, most investigators in the field have in fact demonstrated the capacity of hemoperfusion to reverse coma associated with acute liver failure. In our published studies, 90% of patients awoke [19]. Nevertheless, none of the studies reported are in fact controlled studies thus preventing any solidly based determination of the benefits of hemoperfusion in coma reversal in hepatic failure.

A similar conclusion derives on analysis of data concerning the effects of hemoperfusion on survival of patients with hepatic coma. The study of *Gazzard* et al. [20] in 1974 presented an extremely optimistic view since some 38% of treated patients survived. This was in contrast to previous results by the same group in the same hospital demonstrating approximately 10–15% survival in the same disease without hemoperfusion. Mysteriously, but by no means defying scientific laws of chance variability, a subsequent group of patients treated in a reasonably similar manner faired much less well in the hands of the King's College group. In our hands, approximately 40% of patients treated with charcoal hemoperfusion survived. Again, whether these results are in fact superior to results using any other form of treatment including conservative medical management remains to be presented. There are in fact no controlled clinical trials of which I am aware published to this date. It is unlikely that a single group will derive controlled data but a cooperative undertaking might be successful in determining the answer to this very significant question.

Conclusion

In summary, while considerably more modest, the expectations for hemoperfusion for hepatic failure and the coma associated with hepatic failure have not been particularly well achieved to date. In this entity, because of the peculiar effects on platelets and clotting factors, the hemoperfusion systems currently available are associated with a significant level of complications. Moreover, hepatic coma is an entity wherein the precipitating putative toxin(s) is poorly understood; it is, therefore, difficult to prove the effectiveness of hemoperfusion. Finally, there are virtually no controlled studies wherein the data may be used to substantiate the benefit of hemoperfusion either to reverse coma or to enhance survival in hepatic failure. One can only await controlled trials to define the ultimate role of hemoperfusion.

In conclusion, it might be argued that hemoperfusion in acute hepatic failure might be considered to have achieved the expectations placed upon it if at a minimum this procedure represented the best available therapy. While a considerably less stringent criterion, the argument is a reasonably compelling one. In my estimation, this question should be answered in the affirmative for the vast majority of severe acute toxic ingestions, however, it is extremely difficult to defend the position that hemoperfusion represents the best available therapy for hepatic coma associated with acute hepatic failure. While the available data are certainly suggestive that hemoperfusion is capable of reversing coma, its overall effectiveness and in particular its ability to enhance survival have not been definitively demonstrated.

References

1 Muirhead, E.E.; Reid, A.F.: A resin artificial kidney. J. Lab. clin. Med. *33:* 841–844 (1948).

2 Schreiner, G.E.: The role of hemodialysis (artificial kidney) in acute poisoning. Archs intern. Med. *102:* 896–900 (1958).

3 Hagstam, K.E.; Larsson, L.E.; Thysell, H.: Experimental studies on charcoal haemoperfusion in phenobarbital intoxication and uraemia, including histopathologic findings. Acta med. scand. *180:* 593–603 (1966).

4 Dunea, G.; Kolff, W.J.: Clinical experience with the Yatzidis charcoal. Artif. internal Organs *11:* 178–182 (1965).

5 Yatzidis, H.: A convenient haemoperfusion micro-apparatus over charcoal for the treatment of endogenous and exogenous intoxications. Its use as an artificial kidney. Proc. Eur. Dialysis Transplant. Ass. *1:* 83–87 (1964).

6 Yatzidis, H.; Oreopoulus, D.; Triantaphyllidis, D.; Voudiclari, S.; Tsaparas, N.; Gavras, C.; Stavroulaki, A.: Treatment of severe barbiturate poisoning. Lancet *ii:* 216–217 (1965).

7 Rosenbaum, J.L.; Kramer, M.S.; Raja, R.; Boreyko, C.: Resin hemoperfusion. A new treatment for acute drug intoxication. New Engl. J. Med. *284:* 874–877 (1971).

8 Chang, T.M.S.; Coffey, J.F.; Barre, P.; Gonda, A.; Dirks, J.H.; Levy, M.; Lister, C.: Microcapsule artificial kidney: treatment of patients with acute drug intoxication. Can. med. Ass. J. *17:* 429–433 (1973).

9 Chang, T.M.S.: Hemoperfusion alone and in series with ultrafiltration or dialysis for uremia, poisoning, and liver failure. Kidney int. *10:* 305 (1976).

10 Fennimore, J.; Watson, P.A.; Munro, G.D.; Kolthammer, J.: The design and evaluation of a convenient carbon haemoperfusion system. Proc. Eur. Soc. artif. Organs *1:* 90 (1974).

11 Hill, J.B.; Palaia, F.L.; McAdams, J.L.; Palmer, P.J.; Skinner, J.T.; Maret, S.M.: The rationale for fixed-bed charcoal in hemoperfusion. Kidney int. *10:* 328–332 (1976).

12 Gimson, A.E.S.; Hughes, R.D.; Langley, P.G.; Canalese, J.; Williams, R.: King's experience with artificial liver support; in Sideman, Chang, Hemoperfusion – kidney and liver support and detoxification, pp. 285–293 (Hemisphere Publishing Corp., Washington, D.C., 1980).

13 Gelfand, M.C.: Charcoal hemoperfusion. Georgetown University experience; in Chang, Artificial liver, artificial kidney, and artificial cells, pp. 117–123 (Plenum Press, New York 1978).

14 Bismuth, C.; Conso, F.; Wattel, F.; Gosselin, B.; Lambert, H.; Genestal, M.: Coated activated charcoal hemoperfusion: experience of French antipoison centers about 60 cases. Vet. hum. Toxicol. 21–2 (1979).

15 Medd, R.K.; Widdop, B.; Braithwaite, R.A.; Rees, A.J.; Goulding, R.J.: Comparison of haemoperfusion and haemodialysis on the therapy of barbiturate intoxication in dogs. Archs Toxicol. *31:* 163–174 (1973).

16 Farrell, P.C.: Acute drug intoxication and extracorporeal intervention. Am. Soc. artif. internal Organs *3:* 39–42 (1980).

17 Gibson, T.P.: The pharmacokinetic determinants of the efficacy of hemoperfusion. Workshop of Hemoperfusion, Kidney and Liver Supports and Detoxification 1979.

18 Hampel, G.; Widdop, B.; Goulding, R.: Adsorptive capacity of haemoperfusion devices in clinical use (Abstract). Hemoperfusion, Dialysate, Diafiltrate Purification Symp., Tutzing 1978.

19 Gelfand, M.C.; Knepshield, J.H.; Cohan, S.; Ramirez, B.; Schreiner, G.E.: Treatment of hepatic coma with hemoperfusion through polyacrylamide hydrogen-coated charcoal. Kidney int. *10:* 239–243 (1976).

20 Gazzard, B.G.; Weston, M.J.; Murray-Lyon, I.M.; Flax, H.; Record, C.O.; Portmann, B.; Langley, P.G.; Dunlop, E.H.; Mellon, P.J.; Ward, M.G.; Williams, R.: Charcoal haemoperfusion in the treatment of fulminant hepatic failure. Lancet *i:* 1301–1307 (1974).

21 Clemmesen, C.; Nilsson, E.: Therapeutic trends in the treatment of barbiturate poisoning: the Scandinavian method. Clin. Pharmacol. Ther. *2:* 220 (1961).

22 Lorch, J.A.; Garella, S.: Hemoperfusion to treat intoxications. Ann. intern. Med. *91:* 301 (1979).

23 Zieve, L.: Pathogenesis of hepatic coma. Archs intern. Med. *118:* 211–223 (1966).

24 Lam, K.C.; Tell, A.R.; Goldstein, G.B.: Role of a false neurotransmitter, octopamine, in the pathogenesis of hepatic and renal encephalopathy. Scand. J. Gastroent. *8:* 465–472 (1973).

25 Muto, Y.; Takahashi, Y.J.: Gas chromatographic determination of plasma short-chain fatty acids in diseases of the liver. Jap. Soc. intern. Med. *53:* 828–839 (1964).

26 Hartmann, F.; Lenz, H.: The phenol and indole pattern of rat urine after administration of tyrosine, tryptophan, and phenylalanine and after inhibition of the intestinal flora with neomycin. Dt. Arch. klin. Med. *208:* 29–37 (1962).

27 Challenger, F.; Walshe, J.M.: Methyl mercaptan in relation to foetor hepaticus. Biomed. J. *59:* 3 (1955).

28 Trey, C.; Burns, D.G.; Saunders, S.J.: Treatment of hepatic coma by exchange blood transfusion. New Engl. J. Med. *274:* 473–481 (1966).

29 Fischer, J.E.; Rosen, H.M.; Ebeid, A.M.: The effect of normalization of plasma amino acids on hepatic encephalopathy in man. Surgery *80:* 77–91 (1976).

30 Gelfand, M.C.; Winchester, J.F.; Knepshield, J.H.; Cohan, S.L.; Schreiner, G.E.: Biochemical correlates of reversal of hepatic coma coated with charcoal hemoperfusion. Trans. Am. Soc. artif. internal Organs *24:* 239–242 (1978).

31 Gazzard, B.G.; Weston, M.J.; Murray-Lyon, I.M.: Charcoal haemoperfusion in the treatment of fulminant hepatic failure. Lancet *i:* 1301–1307 (1974).

32 Abouna, G.M.; Barabas, A.Z.; Boyd, N.: Resin and charcoal hemoperfusion in the treatment of hepatic coma; in Kenedi, Courtney, Gaylor, Gilchrist, Artifical organs, p. 363 (Macmillan Press, London 1977).

33 Chen, R.F.: Removal of fatty acids from serum albumin by charcoal treatment. J. biol. Chem. *242:* 173–181 (1967).

34 Holloway, C.J.; Brunner, G.; Schmidt, E.; Schmidt, F.W.: Thiols and hepatic coma. Artif. Organs *3:* 15–19 (1979).

35 Hellwig, G.; Chmiel, H.: Theoretical aspects of adsorption of polar substances from polar solvents. Artif. Organs *3:* 192–193 (1979).

M.C. Gelfand, MD, Georgetown University Medical Center,
Washington, DC 20007 (USA)

Contr. Nephrol., vol. 29, pp. 114–122 (Karger, Basel 1982)

Potential for Hemoperfusion in Uremia

J.F. Winchester[1]
Georgetown University Medical Center, Washington, D.C., USA

Introduction

It is well recognized that while dialytic techniques are of proven value in the treatment of uremia, they carry an appreciable mortality with 10-year survival figures of approximately 50%. The principal cause of death in hemodialysis patients results from cardiovascular catastrophies in over 60% of patients and is thought to result either from persistence of complications of uremia despite dialysis therapy (table I) or complications of dialysis therapy itself. Although initial reports of ion-exchange resin hemoperfusion in animals [1] suggested that urea could be removed from uremic animals, the side effects associated with such treatment were prohibitive and ion-exchange resin hemoperfusion was regarded by many as unsafe [2]. Early reports of charcoal hemoperfusion were also associated with prohibitive side effects since the first charcoal hemoperfusion experiments were carried out with uncoated and poorly washed charcoal. The work of *Chang* [3] with microencapsulation of carbon particles within polymer coating, however, was a stimulus for re-evaluation of hemoperfusion in uremia, but also in other disease states such as poisoning and hepatic coma. It was not surprising that charcoal hemoperfusion by virtue of its nonspecific wide spectrum solute adsorption was one approach that was suggested for the more efficient removal of uremic toxins, and early reports of its use in man have indeed appeared encouraging. It must be pointed out, however, that most of the studies reported have been of a noncritical nature; and it is the purpose of this paper to review the studies in a critical fashion to point out the deficiencies in the studies and also suggest positive avenues for further exploration in the treatment of uremia with hemoperfusion.

[1] I wish to thank both Mrs. *Patti Werr* and Mrs. *Donna Sullivan* for their expert secretarial assistance in preparing this manuscript.

Table I. Complications of uremia persisting with dialysis therapy

Cardiovascular:	refractory hypertension, pericarditis; accelerated atherosclerosis
Dermatological:	pruritus, pigmentation
Endocrine:	lipid abnormalities; protein malnutrition; osteodystrophy thyroid and other endocrine disturbances; infertility; sexual dysfunction
Gastrointestinal:	peptic ulceration
Hematological:	anemia,; platelet dysfunction; leucocyte dysfunction; sepsis; derangements of iron metabolism
Immunological:	decreased immune response
Neurological:	peripheral neuropathy
Pharmacological:	derangements of drug metabolism

Review of Studies

In the last 10 years many studies, predominantly of charcoal hemoperfusion, have been undertaken in the treatment of clinical uremia. These studies have been of a short-term nature (less than 3 months) or of a long-term nature (greater than 3 months) in individual patients. It is estimated that over 150 patients have had some form of hemoperfusion for the treatment of their end-stage renal disease. Several substances thought to be toxic in uremia, and removed by hemoperfusion, are shown in table II, the molecular weight of these substances ranging from 60 to 21,500 daltons. The 'classical' markers of uremia, creatinine, uric acid, indoles, and guanidines, were first reported to be removed by charcoal hemoperfusion in 1964 by *Yatzidis* [4]. The removal of these substances has been confirmed with the use of uncoated activated charcoal hemoperfusion [4–8] and also for coated charcoal hemoperfusion [9–14]. More recently attention has been directed to the removal of other substances such as amino acids [11, 12, 14] and hormones [12, 14]. It has been thought for some time that the 'middle molecule' hypothesis explains most of the features of intractable uremia, despite dialysis therapy, and several authors have reported that charcoal hemoperfusion removes considerable quantities of middle molecules [10–12, 14], although in the study by *Oules* et al. [11] there was variable removal of middle molecules with rapid uptake at the initiation of hemoperfusion but saturation of the sorbent for middle molecules thereafter.

Short-term studies of hemoperfusion in uremia have defined the necessary prerequisites for hemoperfusion in uremia, namely (1) sufficient sorbent uptake of putative uremic toxins; (2) safety; (3) reversal of some features of uremia.

Table II. Uremic toxins removed by sorbents (MW 60–21,500 daltons)

Adrenocorticotrophin	(Myoinositol)
(Aldosterone)	Non-protein nitrogen
Amino acids	Nor-epinephrine
Calcium	Organic acids
25, OH-cholecalciferol	Oxalate
Creatinine	Parathyroid Hormone
Cyclic AMP	Phenols
Epinephrine	(Phosphate)
Folic acid	Polyamino acids
Gastrin	(Renin)
Glucagon	Ribonuclease
Glucose	Serotonin
(Growth hormone)	Thyroxine
Guanidines	Trace metals; As, Co, Cr, Se
Indoles	Triglycerides
Insulin	Triiodothyronine
L-Dopamine	(Urea)
(Magnesium)	Uric acid
Middle molecules	Vitamin B_{12}

() = Poorly removed.

Long-term studies, on the other hand, have used the data from the short-term studies (particularly on safety) and have concentrated on reversal of some aspects of uremia such as peripheral neuropathy and pericarditis.

The effects of hemoperfusion in uremia have been reviewed in depth by *Winchester* [15, 16]. All the studies have attested to the fact that urea, water, and electrolytic substances are not removed by hemoperfusion and most modern studies use a combination of hemoperfusion with dialysers or with ultrafiltration devices.

Biochemical Changes with Short- and Long-Term Hemoperfusion

The clinical studies reported have not been uniformly consistent in their choice of sorbents, the quantity of sorbent used in the devices, the blood flow rate through the devices, etc. For sake of clarity in comparing the studies, I have chosen to adjust the reported data in the studies to a uniform value. I have chosen to report initial solute clearances (usually after 15 min of hemoperfusion alone or with hemodialysis) per gram of sorbent, adjusted to a blood flow rate of 300 ml/min. These values are reported in tables III and IV. It is apparent that uncoated charcoal possesses a higher initial solute clearance than coated char-

Table III. Initial solute clearance (ml/min/g sorbent) adjusted for blood flow rate 300 ml/min

Short- and long-term studies	Uncoated charcoal				
	creatinine	urate	phenols	guanidines	indoles
Yatzidis, 1964 [4]	1.32	1.36	1.05	1.14	1.14
Dunea and Kolff, 1965 [5]	1.2				
Dunea et al., 1975 [6] (HP/HD)	1.5				
Siemsen et al., 1978 [7] (HP/HD)	1.5				
Rosenbaum et al., 1980 [8] (HP/HD)	1.32	1.32			

HP/HD = Hemoperfusion/hemodialysis.

Table IV. Initial solute clearance (ml/min/g sorbent) adjusted for blood flow rate 300 ml/min

Short- and long-term studies	Coated charcoal					
	creatinine	urate	phenols	homones	amino acids	middle molecules
Chang et al., 1971 [9]	0.8	0.9				
Chang, 1976 [10] (HP/HD)	0.72	0.68				0.44
Oules et al., 1977 [11]	0.9	0.9			+	+
Winchester et al., 1978 [12] (HP)	0.6	0.4		+	+	+
(HP/HD)	0.9	0.55		+	+	+
Martin et al., 1978 [13]	0.8	0.8	0.49			
Stefoni et al., 1980 [14] (HP)	0.77	0.55				0.31
(HP/HD)	1.74	1.19				0.52

coal, although this value fails to underscore the common observation that uncoated charcoal saturates rapidly for solutes while coated charcoal has a slower initial uptake but in general a larger total capacity. For coated charcoal hemoperfusion, however, there is a reduction in initial solute clearance occasioned by the thickness of the coating membrane. This is particularly seen in the studies of

Winchester et al. [12] and *Stefoni* et al. [14] where there is a substantial difference in the clearance of solutes with hemoperfusion compared to combined hemoperfusion-hemodialysis treatment. However, the results reported in table IV show that, in general, solute clearance does not differ too much between devices used in these studies.

Safety

Uncoated activated charcoal was largely abandoned because of the profound platelet depletion seen with the early devices [4, 5]. However, introduction of the Hemodetoxifier® (Becton Dickinson, USA) which utilized uncoated carbon fixed to a polyethylene sheet and wound in a spiral has been used in short-term [6] and long-term studies [7]. This device can be associated with profound platelet depletion if the device is primed with a dextran solution [7], but is generally associated with a 30–40% platelet fall. These devices are also notable for removal of calcium and glucose, although this can occasionally occur during coated charcoal hemoperfusion. Of all the coated charcoal hemoperfusion devices, the two devices that stand as the most biocompatible are those of *Chang* [10] which utilized albumin collodion-coated activated charcoal granules and that of *Stefoni* et al. [14] which utilizes extruded activated charcoal coated with a methacrylic hydrogel. Other devices produce an approximately 30% fall in platelet count [12].

It remains to be seen whether the long-term effects of hormone removal [12, 14, 17] and that of trace metal removal [18] will have any bearing on depletion states induced by hemoperfusion. *Chang* et al. [19] have shown that residual blood volume of the devices is 7.0 ml and *Stefoni* et al. [14] have shown with their devices' residual blood volume is 3.1 ml. This strongly contrasts with the blood loss of 100 ml with each use of the uncoated charcoal devices reported initially by *Dunea and Kolff* [5]. In summary, for repetitive use it would appear that charcoal hemoperfusion is indeed safe for study in chronic uremia.

Reversal of Uremic Symptomatology

Short-term studies have shown that several symptoms of uremia can be reversed by the application of charcoal hemoperfusion. These are pericarditis [4, 20] but also gastrointestinal symptoms and lethargy [9, 10]. On the other hand, it has been shown in the long-term studies of *Chang* et al. [19], *Otsubo* et al. [21], *Agishi* et al. [22] and *Stefoni* et al. [14] that considerable improvement occurs in peripheral neuropathy. In addition, *Stefoni* et al. [14] have shown that other symptoms of uremia such as pruritus and pericarditis are considerably reduced in frequency when hemoperfusion is applied during a long period of time along with hemodialysis. In addition, the exciting report of *Stefoni* et al. [14] of reduction of blood urea nitrogen (BUN) with long-term hemoperfusion may suggest that the protein catabolic rate is being reduced during the period of hemoperfusion. It must also be pointed out, however, that according to *Henderson and Kennedy* [personal communication, 1981] who have employed thrice weekly hemoperfusion with Sutcliffe-Speakman charcoal, 100 g, coated with acrylic hydrogel, along with hemodialysis for 9 months in 9 patients, this treatment has not been associated with a change in mean nerve conduction velocity.

Discussion

The most significant outcome of the extant studies (short- or long-term) has been that charcoal hemoperfusion appears to be relatively safe for the treatment of uremia. What has not yet been demonstrated is its definitive role in the treatment of specific complications of uremia of any significant advantage over standard hemodialysis. In terms of solute removal, however, there appears to be more middle molecule removal, although small molecule removal with a short (2–4 h) combined hemoperfusion/hemodialysis falls short of that achieved with a standard hemodialysis of 5 hours' duration [12]. Moreover, the studies do lack 'tight' control over trial design.

The design of any trial of hemoperfusion in uremia is hampered by several factors. First, a specific sorbent system to adsorb known uremic toxins is not yet feasible since it would appear that the toxins are not directly linked to producing uremic complications, are of wide-ranging biochemical character, and uremic toxicity is probably multifactorial in origin [23]. Secondly, although animal models do exist for production of short-term uremia, no 'true' animal model of chronic human uremia exists. Thirdly, the extant hemoperfusion studies already undertaken in uremia differ in the quantities of sorbents chosen for the different devices and differ in the total adsorbent capacity of the devices. Moreover, rarely has residual renal function, in terms of glomerular filtration rate been reported, although *Chang* et al. [19] and *Stefoni* et al. [14] have reported residual renal function in their patients. The important observation by *Stefoni* et al. [14] that BUN appeared to fall over the treatment period with intermittent hemoperfusion in conjunction with hemodialysis suggests that either protein intake is curtailed spontaneously by the patients because of symptoms during the treatment period, or that indeed protein catabolic rates and urea generation rates are improved because of removal of unknown toxic factors. It must be pointed out, however, that no study has addressed urea generation rate or protein catabolic rate changes during the addition of hemoperfusion to hemodialysis.

The most important criticism of all of the studies including my own has been that they have been, of necessity, of 'open' design. In view of the important observations in the short-term of improvement in pericarditis, and in the long-term of reported improvements in nerve conduction velocities, in order to gain acceptance in the dialysis community, it must be shown in a double-blind fashion that hemoperfusion significantly improves these severe complications of uremia. Unlike studies in hepatic failure, it should be eminently feasible to undertake double-blind controlled studies of hemoperfusion in uremia in view of the large number of patients already being treated in the world for end-stage renal disease.

The optimal 'study' of hemoperfusion in uremia should be of a double-blind nature. It should assess changes in mean nerve conduction velocity, it should assess the alteration in frequency and severity of pruritus and pericarditis and lack of well-being. In addition to measurements of glomerular filtration rates on a frequent basis, the opportunity should also be taken to measure urea generation and protein catabolic rates. In addition to the double-blind study, I also suggest that prolonged combined hemoperfusion/hemodialysis patients should be directly compared to a well-matched control group undergoing standard hemodialysis to assess the frequency of uremic symptomatology and objective uremic complications, and also to assess such parameters as trace metal removal and hormone removal.

Since hemoperfusion does not remove urea, water, and electrolytes of necessity, it will have to be combined with hemodialysis or ultrafiltration and additionally several authors have suggested that hemoperfusion combine not only sorption of the solutes such as creatinine and urate but also should attempt to adsorb classical 'markers' of uremia such as urea [24].

The observations on pericarditis and peripheral neuropathy are so important to the management of patients with clinical uremia that it behoves us to prove in an acceptable scientific fashion for the medical community at large that hemoperfusion is of any value in uremic toxicity. The time is now ripe for setting up a controlled clinical study of hemoperfusion in addition to hemodialysis whether of a national or international nature, and I urge that this be undertaken within the near future.

Summary

Despite the introduction of hemoperfusion with resins for uremia in 1948, sorbent hemoperfusion for the treatment of uremia has not yet occupied a place in the routine clinical treatment of end-stage renal disease. Ion-exchange resins for the removal of suspected uremic toxins have largely been abandoned, since they possess prohibitive clinical side effects, and studies have revolved principally around the use of activated charcoal hemoperfusion. Short-term studies of activated charcoal hemoperfusion in uremic patients have shown that coated charcoal hemoperfusion is most biocompatible, and coated charcoal hemoperfusion devices possess adequate capability for adsorbing creatinine, uric acid, guanidines, indoles, phenols, and 'middle molecular weight' substances (although in the latter regard, studies have reported variable adsorption of these middle molecules). It has been clearly demonstrated that charcoal hemoperfusion does not possess the ability to remove water, urea, and electrolyte substances and hemoperfusion requires combination with hemodialysis or ultrafiltration apparatus to achieve removal of these substances. Short-term clinical studies of charcoal hemoperfusion have demonstrated resolution of pericarditis principally, but also improvement in pruritus and lethargy. On the other hand, long-term studies have demonstrated improvement in mean nerve conduction velocity (although this is not invariable) and reduction in frequency of pruritus, pericarditis, and asthenia. All of the studies, however, suffer from the lack of a controlled prospective format, and are hampered by the impossibility of designing specific toxin-removing devices since the 'uremic toxin' is unknown and all require combination with dialysis systems. It is suggested that the time is now ripe for a controlled clinical study (in a double-blind fashion with sham hemoperfusion devices) of the application of hemoperfusion to specific complications occurring during hemodialysis, particularly peripheral neuropathy and pericarditis. Since open studies of hemoperfusion have suggested that pericarditis and peripheral neuropathy are significantly improved, in view of the importance of these observations, it is now imperative that we seek scientific confirmation of the observations.

References

1 Muirhead, E.E.; Reid, A.F.: Resin artificial kidney. J. Lab. clin. Med. *33:* 841–844 (1948).

2 Rosenbaum, J.L.; Onesti, G.; Heider, C.: The removal of cation from dogs with an ion-exchange column. J. Am. med. Ass. *180:* 762–763 (1962).

3 Chang, T.M.S.: Semipermeable aquaeous microcapoules (artificial cells): with emphasis on experiments in an extracorporeal shunt system. Trans. Am. Soc. artif. internal Organs *12:* 13–19 (1966).

4 Yatzidis, H.: A convenient haemoperfusion micro-apparatus over charcoal for the treatment of endogenous and exogenous intoxications. Its use as an artificial kidney. Proc. Eur. Dial. Transpl. Ass. *1:* 83–87 (1964).

5 Dunea, G.; Kolff, W.J.: Clinical experiences with the Yatzidis charcoal artificial kidney. Trans. Am. Soc. artif. internal Organs *11:* 178–182 (1965).

6 Dunea, G.; Rizvi, Z.H.; Mamdani, B.H.; Anicama, H.J.; Mahurkar, S.D.: Charcoal hemoperfusion and combination dialysis-hemoperfusion in chronic renal failure. Abstr. Am. Soc. artif. internal Organs *5:* 22 (1975).

7 Siemsen, A.W.; Dunea, G.; Mamdani, B.H.; Guruprakash, G.: Charcoal hemoperfusion for chronic renal failure. Nephron *22:* 386–390 (1978).

8 Rosenbaum, J.L.; Kramer, M.S.; Raja, R.; Henriquez, M.: Hemoperfusion in uremia: effect of time, solute competition, and biocompatibility on column adsorption; in Sideman, Chang, Hemoperfusion, kidney, and liver support, and detoxification, pp. 245–254 (Hemisphere Publishing, Washington 1980).

9 Chang, T.M.S.; Gonda, A.; Dirks, J.H.; Malave, N.: Clinical evaluation of chronic intermittent and short term hemoperfusion in patients with chronic renal failure using semipermeable microcapsules (artificial cells) formed from membrane coated activated charcoal. Trans. Am. Soc. artif. internal Organs *17:* 246–252 (1971).

10 Chang, T.M.S.: Hemoperfusion alone and in series with ultrafiltration or dialysis for uremia, poisoning, and liver failure. Kidney Int., suppl. 10 pp. 305–311 (1976).

11 Oules, R.; Asaba, H.; Neuhauser, M.; Yahiel, V.; Gunnarsson, B.; Bergstrom, J.; Furst, P.: Removal of uremic small and middle molecules and free amino acids by carbon hemoperfusion. Trans. Am. Soc. artif. internal Organs *23:* 583–589 (1977).

12 Winchester, J.F.; Ratcliffe, J.G.; Carlyle, E.; Kennedy, A.C.: Solute, amino acid, and hormone changes with coated charcoal hemoperfusion in uremia. Kidney Int. *14:* 74–81 (1978).

13 Martin, A.M.; Gibbins, J.K.; Oduro, M.; Herbert, R.: Clinical experience with cellulose coated carbon hemoperfusion; Chang, Artificial liver, artificial kidney, and artificial cells, p. 143 (Plenum Press, New York 1978).

14 Stefoni, S.; Coli, L.; Feliciangeli, G.; Baldrati, L.; Bonomini, V.: Regular hemoperfusion in regular dialysis treatment. A long-term study. Int. J. artif. Organs *3:* 348–353 (1980).

15 Winchester, J.F.: Hemoperfusion in uremia; in Giordano, Sorbents and their clinical applications, p. 387 (Academic Press, New York 1980).

16 Winchester, J.F.: Hemoperfusion; in Drukker, Parson, Maher, Replacement of renal function by dialysis: 2nd ed. (Martinus Nijhoff Publishers, The Hague in press).

17 Kokot, F.; Pietrek, J.; Seredynski, M.: Influence of haemoperfusion on plasma levels of hormone and β-methyldigoxin. Proc. Eur. Dial. Transpl. Ass. *15:* 604–606 (1978).

18 Cornelis, R.; Ringoir, S.; Mees, L.; Hoste, J.: Behavior of trace metals during hemoperfusion. Mineral Electrolyte Metab. *4:* 123–129 (1980).

19 Chang, T.M.S.; Chirito, E.; Barre, B.; Cole, C.; Hewish, M.: Clinical performance-characteristics of a new combined system for simultaneous hemoperfusion-hemodialysis-ultrafiltration in series. Trans. Am. Soc. artif. internal Organs *21:* 502–508 (1975).

20 Martin, A.M.; Gibbins, J.K.; Kimmit, J.; Rennie, F.: Hemodialysis and hemoperfusion in the treatment of uremic pericarditis. A study of 13 cases. Dial. Transpl. *8:* 135–136 (1979).

21 Otsubo, O.; Kuzuhara, K.; Simada, Y.; Yamauchi, Y.; Takahashi, I.; Yamada, Y.; Otsubo, K.; Inou, T.: Treatment of uraemic peripheral neuritis by direct haemoperfusion with activated charcoal. Proc. Eur. Dial. Transpl. Ass. *16:* 731–736 (1979).

22 Agishi, T.; Yamashita, N.; Ota, K.: Clinical results of direct charcoal hemoperfusion for endogenous and exogenous intoxication; in Sideman, Chang, Hemoperfusion, kidney, and liver support and detoxification, p. 255 (Hemisphere Publishing Corp., Washington 1980).

23 Schreiner, G.E.; Winchester, J.F.: Uremia – 1978 perspective. Clin. Nephrol. *11:* 52 (1979).

24 Winchester, J.F.; Gelfand, M.C.; Knepshield, J.H.; Schreiner, G.E.: Realities in evaluating the clinical uses of sorbent hemoperfusion. Int. J. artif. Organs *2:* 310–314 (1979).

J.F. Winchester, MD, Georgetown University Medical Center,
Washington, DC 20007 (USA)

Contr. Nephrol., vol. 29, pp. 123–132 (Karger, Basel 1982)

Use of Combined Hemodialysis/Hemoperfusion in Chronic Uremia[1]

S. Stefoni, G. Feliciangeli, L. Colì, R. Prandini, V. Bonomini
Institute of Nephrology and Dialysis, University of Bologna, Italy

Introduction

In hemoperfusion direct contact is achieved between the blood and particles of material (sorbent) capable of absorbing molecules retained or introduced exogenously. The characteristic of an ideal sorbent should include, in addition to effectiveness in removing 'toxins', safety and capacity of not removing from the blood molecules, structures and cells of biological value.

Activated charcoal has been shown to be an effective sorbent for many drugs and waste metabolism. Its therapeutic use has long been limited to oral ingestion, which is fairly effective in a very limited number of conditions. More recently activated charcoal granules have been used by several authors for hemoperfusion in patients with chronic renal failure [6, 8, 16, 17], hepatic coma [5, 11, 18] and intoxication [4, 19]. Since the first experience it has been shown that uncoated charcoal releases microemboli, while its poor biocompatibility results in severe platelet and blood cell depletion [7]. These drawbacks have been significantly overcome by coating the granules of charcoal with various membranes which slightly reduce the sorption capacity but highly increase the biocompatibility of the charcoal. The thickness and characteristics of coating membranes available today are described elsewhere in this issue [9].

Charcoal Hemoperfusion in Uremia

The introduction of hemodialysis therapy has allowed patients affected by chronic renal failure to survive. The increasing influx of patients to regular dialysis treatment combined with a higher survival rate has given rise, among other things, to two problems: (1) improvement of the patient's quality of life and as

[1] Supported in part by Italian CNR grant No. CT 80.00388.04.

full a rehabilitation as possible; (2) finding the most efficient purifying processes possible, to cope with treating a growing number of patients by means of the same facilities.

Despite its wide application and its effectiveness dialysis remains an unphysiological way of treatment. The metabolic and endocrine functions of the intact kidney are not substituted: the patient is machine-dependent; many uremic signs persist or worsen as the years on dialysis go by and some dialysis-related diseases can also appear. Several medical and technological approaches have been suggested to improve the overall clinical results of long-term dialysis. Medical approaches include early dialysis [2]; physical exercise [21]; hormone and drug therapy; trace metals control; diet and others. Today's technological potential is high. Its development and clinical application, however, must always consider the patients' needs and characteristics. The most recent advances in renal technology include the use of highly permeable membranes [10], the introduction of new schedules, hemofiltration [22], new dialysates, bicarbonate, miniaturization of apparatus, alternative ways of treatment [24], hemoperfusion and others.

Charcoal hemoperfusion might play an important role in this field. The proven capacity of activated charcoal to remove endogenous and exogenous toxins from the blood strongly suggests the validity of charcoal use in uremia, where a whole range of 'toxic' substances is retained in the body. Charcoal hemoperfusion in chronic uremia has long been proposed and applied by several authors [6, 17, 20, 23] as an adjunct, alternative or substitute for hemodialysis.

The major drawbacks to its regular use in the treatment of uremic patients have been: (1) poor biocompatibility of charcoal; (2) its inability to remove water, electrolytes, urea and phosphate, and (3) its cost. Biocompatibility is extremely important where long-term treatment of patients is concerned. While capable of removing creatinine, uric acid and other substances up to a molecular weight of 10,000–12,000 daltons, charcoal is unable to remove urea, electrolytes and water. In the long-term treatment of uremic patients it thus becomes necessary to plan the use of hemoperfusion in association with ultrafiltration, hemofiltration or hemodialysis. Lastly, the problem of cost must be considered carefully.

The experience of our group in the use of hemoperfusion in uremic patients followed several phases: (1) procuring reliable coated charcoal devices; (2) evaluation of biocompatibility and tolerance; (3) efficiency evaluation, and (4) clinical application.

Hemoperfusion Device

Since 1977 we have used a hemoperfusion apparatus containing activated charcoal coated with a new methacrylate-based membrane of improved biocompatibility (Biotec Hemoperfusion System). The characteristics of the device have

Table I. Side effects observed during combined HD/HP treatment (total procedures = 520)

Side effects	n	Sessions interrupted
Nausea	2	–
Muscular cramp	3	–
Headache	3	–
Chills	15	5
Fever	8	2
Hypotension	6	1

previously been described [13]. The charcoal content of the cartridge was initially 300 g. Later on in the programme of regular combination of hemoperfusion with hemodialysis (see below) the quantity of charcoal was reduced to 150 g.

Coating Membrane. The coating membrane is 1.5 μm thick and utilizes hydroxyethylmethacrylate as a basic element. When suitably cross-linked, this forms a copolymer in block form, in which the hydrophilic block has the property of swelling and division, while the hydrophobe block contributes a mechanical resistance to the moist membrane. It is known that water content and molecular structure play an important role in determining the permeability and the biocompatibility of hydrogels. Methacrylate membranes have already been used for coating activated charcoal [1]. Results have not been completely satisfactory (mainly because of platelet depletion and aggregation) possibly due to the scanty uniformity of the coating and to the rather low hydrophilic action of the hydrogel (40% water absorption) by weight [1]. We used a coating membrane affording 60% water absorption. Hydrophilia was increased by copolymerization of hydroxyethylmethacrylate with an unsaturated heterocyclical compound that is highly hydrophilic in the presence of appropriate cross-links. The expected deterioration of the mechanical properties was minimized by introducing within the tridimensional polymeric network a fourth monomer with hydrophobic and elastomeric properties [12].

Biocompatibility and Tolerance

The biocompatibility and tolerance of a hemoperfusion device are of primary importance where long-term treatment is concerned. In vitro and in vivo studies demonstrated that the biocompatibility of the methacrylate-coated charcoal can be regarded as highly satisfactory [13]. As for tolerance, table I shows the main side effects found in 520 combined hemodialysis/hemoperfusion (HD/HP) sessions.

Efficiency

The efficiency of the methacrylate-coated charcoal was evaluated in vivo and in vitro by measuring the sorption capacity of substances of increasing molecular weight (urea, creatinine, uric acid, digoxin, vitamin B_{12}, lysozyme). The varying clearance rate with time of perfusion was also evaluated [14]. The smaller quantity of charcoal contained in the cartridge we used (150 g) afforded rather low clearance of small molecules (less than 200 daltons) compared with standard dialyzers and other 300-gram charcoal cartridges. However, for substances of greater molecular size (up to 2,000 daltons) the reduced quantitiy of charcoal seems to ensure an equally satisfactory removal. Methacrylate-coated charcoal has a capacity, albeit limited, for removing substances of molecular weight of up to about 14,000 daltons. The overall long-term effects of the combined HD/HP program were evaluated by clinical, hematochemical and instrumental investigations [14].

Clinical Application

As is known, charcoal hemoperfusion is capable of removing many uremic toxins, but is incapable of removing urea, electrolytes and water. In chronic uremia, therefore, hemoperfusion must be combined with dialysis or ultrafiltration, if a long-term treatment is planned. The combined HD/HP session has been the basis of our schedule of treatment. In such sessions (fig. 1) a cartridge containing 150 g of activated charcoal is inserted in the dialysis circuit in series with the dialyzer, flat plate or hollow fiber. The cartridge is left in situ throughout the whole session. As a rule the circuit is rinsed with 1,500 ml of normal saline, containing 30,000 IU of heparin. The patient is connected to the circuit without wasting the priming volume. The further amount of heparin needed for the HD/HP procedure is generally the same as that used in hemodialysis alone. The care required by the staff for the HD/HP procedure is similar to that for dialysis alone.

HD/HP Program

The HD/HP program involves substituting one or more of the weekly dialysis sessions with one or more combined HD/HP procedures. The aims of the HD/HP program were the clinical and metabolic improvement of patients and/or the reduction of the weekly time of treatment. The combined HD/HP treatment was employed in three groups of informed patients on regular dialysis, who volunteered to take part in the program. Throughout the study all patients followed their previous dietary and drug regimen unchanged.

Group 1 included 13 patients with persisting or recurring signs of uremia despite technically adequate dialysis, as regards time of treatment, blood flow,

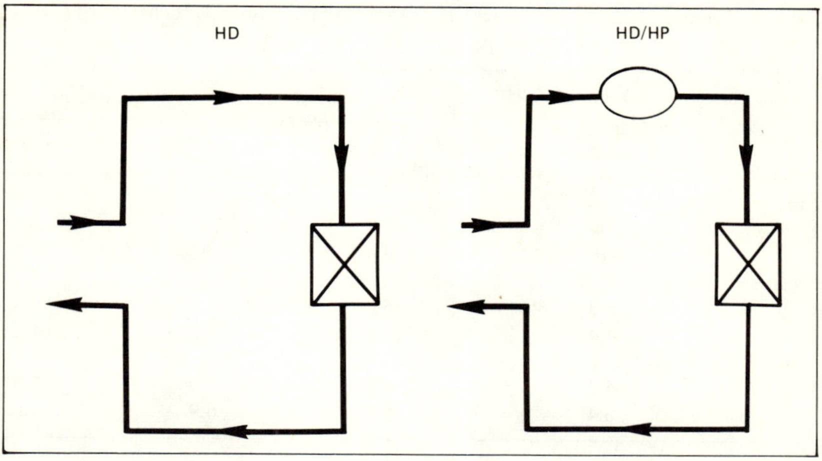

Fig. 1. Combined HD/HP procedure.

dialyzer efficiency, etc. In this group the aim of the HD/HP treatment was the clinical improvement of patients. They mainly complained of pruritus, recurring fibrinous pericarditis, severe peripheral neuropathy, gastrointestinal symptoms and asthenia. A general lack of well-being was reported by all patients. In these patients one combined HD/HP procedure took the place of one of the weekly hemodialysis procedures. Treatment lasted from 4 to 51 weeks. The regular combination of hemoperfusion and dialysis resulted in disappearance of most dialysis-resistant uremic signs. In 8 patients who underwent treatment for at last 13 weeks without interruption we found a 14.8% decrease in plasma creatinine, a 25.6% decrease in uric acid and a 19.8% decrease in plasma urea. All decreases were statistically significant [14]. Motor nerve conduction velocity, which was very low at the beginning of treatment, increased markedly, although not to a statistically significant degree.

Group 2 included 5 patients on dialysis which was both technically and clinically adequate. 3 patients were on three dialyses per week, 2 on two dialyses per week. In this group the aim of the HD/HP program was to investigate the possibility of reducing the weekly time of treatment. Here in all patients one combined HD/HP session replaced two hemodialysis sessions of the previous hemodialysis schedule. Despite this marked reduction in hours of treatment, clinical and metabolic conditions remained unchanged. In this group too the tolerance of treatment was good. However, it must be admitted that this group of patients was rather selective: all patients had diuresis, and their mean residual creatinine clearance was 7 ml/min [2]. We accordingly studied a third group of patients.

Table II. Combined HD/HP treatment in chronic uremia (group 3): behavior of urea, creatinine and uric acid (mg%ml) in two patients

Patient No.	Before HD/HP	After		
		1 month	3 months	5 months
Urea				
1	184	166	210	215
2	210	204	195	219
Creatinine				
1	13.3	15.0	16.7	16.0
2	14.4	15.0	15.3	14.2
Urate				
1	6.2	6.8	7.9	7.5
2	6.4	5.9	6.9	6.6

Group 3 included 5 patients with a mean residual creatinine clearance of 1.8 and a mean diuresis of 350 ml on dialysis (three times/week), which was again both technically and clinically adequate. As in group 2 the aim of the HD/HP treatment was to reduce the time of treatment. The study lasted from 13 to 31 weeks and the treatment still continues. As for the schedule, two combined HD/HP sessions abruptly replaced the three previous dialysis sessions. In these patients the net and actual reduction in time of treatment was therefore 33%. To evaluate the results and the tolerance of the HD/HP treatment we considered clinical, metabolic and hematochemical parameters. Table II shows the behavior with time of plasma creatinine, uric acid and urea in the 2 anuric patients in a 5-month period of treatment. It can be said that all parameters remained unchanged or increased very slightly despite the 33% reduction in time of treatment. Tolerance: fibrinogen (fig. 2), platelets (fig. 3) and white cells (fig. 4) remained unchanged throughout treatment. From a clinical point of view the conditions of patients remained unchanged: personal, family and social rehabilitation was, of course, improved. The complete analysis of all long-term results obtained in these patients is undergoing evaluation [15].

Conclusions

The high biocompatibility of many coating membranes today available, including the new methacrylate-based membrane we used, allows a long-term charcoal hemoperfusion in chronic uremia. The combination of dialysis with hemoperfusion gets round some intrinsic limits of charcoal, while the regular

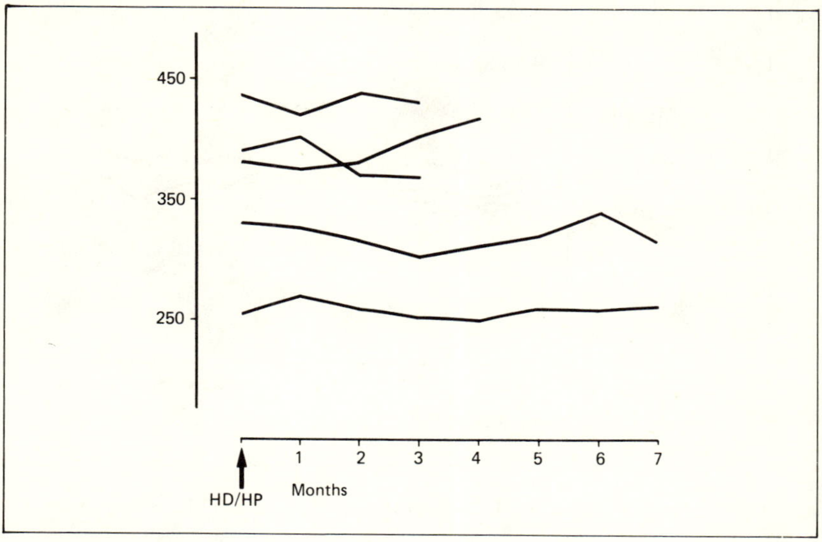

Fig. 2. Long-term combined HD/HP treatment. Effects on fibrinogen (mg%ml).

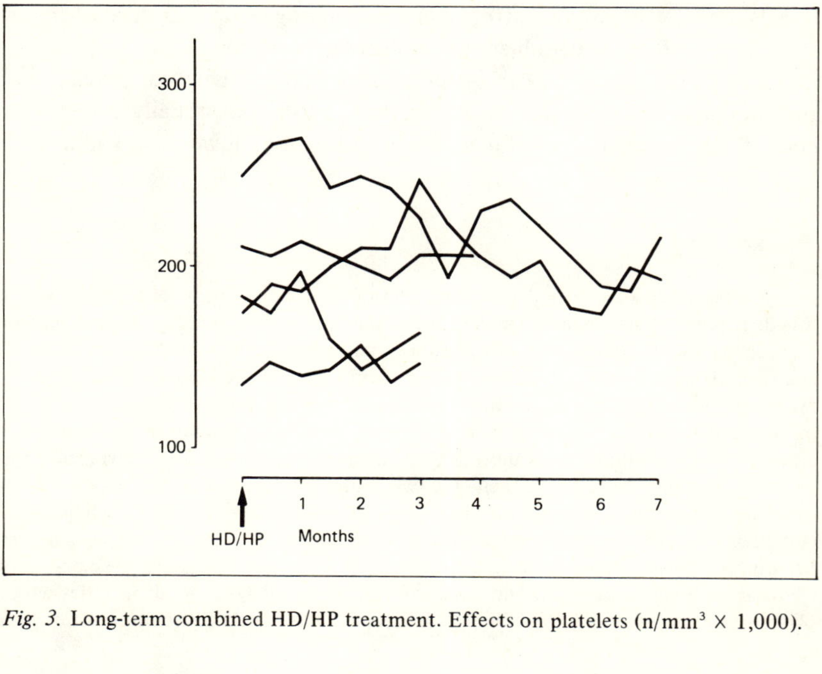

Fig. 3. Long-term combined HD/HP treatment. Effects on platelets (n/mm^3 × 1,000).

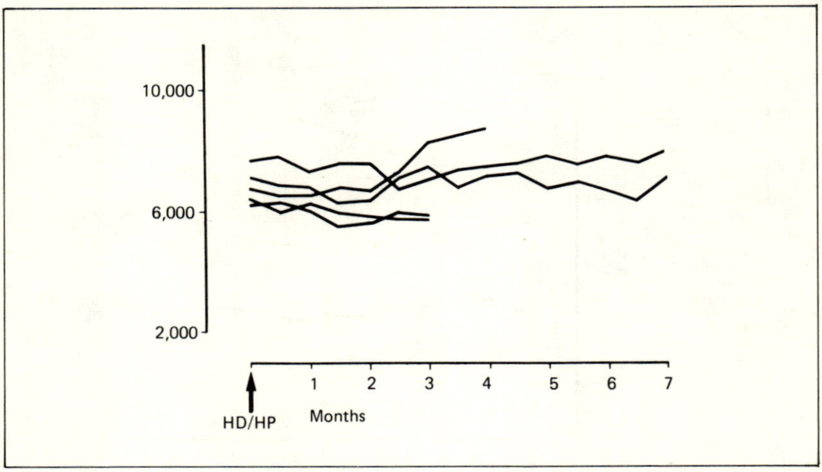

Fig. 4. Long-term combined HD/HP treatment. Effects on white cells (n/mm^3).

combination of hemoperfusion with dialysis leads to the disappearance of a series of dialysis-resistant uremic signs (group 1 patients). In other patients (groups 2 and 3) the HD/HP program affords an actual saving of up to a third of the overall treatment time, without subjective or objective worsening.

Lastly, the use of a cartridge containing 150 g of charcoal instead of 300 g, together with the reduction in dialysis time per week, partially offsets the high cost of the charcoal. A careful economic evaluation, however, is still needed [3].

Summary

The capacity of charcoal to absorb endogenous and exogenous toxins is well established. It removes substances of higher molecular weight than standard dialysis membranes. The regular use of charcoal hemoperfusion as an adjunct to hemodialysis in chronic uremia is a real prospect capable of improving the patient's clinical and laboratory condition and/or reducing the weekly time of treatment. In line with our previous experience, 5 consenting informed patients on regular dialysis treatment from 9 to 35 months (residual creatinine clearance 0–1.8 ml/min, mean diuresis 350 ml) were treated without interruption for 5–8 months according to a schedule including two combined hemodialysis/hemoperfusion procedures instead of the previous three hemodialysis sessions. Patients were on adequate dialysis and their clinical, metabolic and laboratory conditions were stable. In the hemodialysis/hemoperfusion procedure a cartridge containing 150 g of methacrylate-coated activated charcoal with high biocompatibility was inserted in the dialysis circuit in series with a flat plate or hollow fiber dialyzer. Clinical, laboratory and metabolic conditions remained unchanged in all patients despite the one third reduction in dialysis hours per week. The tolerance of treatment was good: platelets, white cells and fibrinogen were unaffected. The marked reduction in weekly time of treatment led to a more satisfactory personal and social rehabilitation, enabling more patients to be treated with the same facilities.

References

1 Andrade, J.D.; Kunitomo, K.; van Wagener, R.; Kastigir, B.; Gough, D.; Kolff, W.J.: Coated adsorbents for direct blood perfusion: HEMA/activated carbon. Trans. Am. Soc. artif. internal Organs *17:* 222 (1971).

2 Bonomini, V.: Early dialysis 1979. Nephron *24:* 157 (1979).

3 Bonomini, V.; Zanetti, M.: Cost/benefit analysis of long-term hemodialysis/hemoperfusion treatment in chronic uremia (1981).

4 Chang, T.M.S.: Removal of endogenous and exogenous toxins by a microencapsulated adsorbent. Can. J. Physiol. Pharmacol. *47:* 1,043 (1969).

5 Chang, T.M.S.: Hemoperfusion over microencapsulated adsorbent in a patient with hepatic coma. Lancet *ii:* 1371 (1972).

6 Chang, T.M.S.: Hemoperfusion alone and in series with ultrafiltration or dialysis for uremia, poisoning and liver failure. Kidney int. *10:* 305 (1976).

7 Chang, T.M.S.: Protective effects of microencapsulated coating on platelet depletion and particulate embolism in the clinical application of charcoal hemoperfusion; in Artificial organs, pp. 164–177 (Macmillan Press, London 1977).

8 Chang, T.M.S.: Assessments of clinical trials of charcoal hemoperfusion in uremic patients. Clin. Nephrol. *11:* 111 (1979).

9 Chang, T.M.S.: Hemoperfusion in 1981 (this issue, 1981).

10 Funck-Brentano, J.L.; Man, N.K.; Sausse, A.: Effect of more porous dialysis membrane on neuropathic toxins. Kidney int. *7:* 52 (1974).

11 Gazzard, B.G.; Portman, B.A.; Weston, M.J.; Langley, P.G.; Murray-Lyon, I.M.; Dunlop, E.M.; Flax, H.; Mellon, P.J.; Record, C.O.; Ward, M.B.; Williams, R.: Charcoal hemoperfusion in the treatment of fulminant hepatic failure. Lancet *i:* 1301 (1974).

12 Plicchi, G.; Betti, V.; Canducci, G.C.; Pagani, P.; Rossi, M.; Spighi, M.; Zingaretti, G.: Study and evaluation of a new hydrophilic polymer for the coating of activated carbons for hemoperfusion. Policlinico, Sez. chir. *84:* 37 (1977).

13 Stefoni, S.; Feliciangeli, G.; Colì, L.; Bonomini, V.: Evaluation of a new coated charcoal for hemoperfusion in uremia. Int. J. artif. Organs *2:* 320 (1979).

14 Stefoni, S.; Colì, L.; Feliciangeli, G.; Baldrati, L.; Bonomini, V.: Regular hemoperfusion in regular dialysis treatment. A long-term study. Int. J. artif. Organs *3:* 348 (1980).

15 Stefoni, S.; Colì, L.; Feliciangeli, G.; Bonomini, V.: Combined hemodialysis/hemoperfusion treatment as a mean to reduce the weekly hours of treatment in RDT patients. Int. J. artif. Organs, *4:* 186 (1981).

16 Winchester, J.F.; Apiliga, M.T.; Mackay, J.M.; Kennedy, A.C.: Hemodialysis with charcoal hemoperfusion. Proc. Eur. Dialysis Transplant. Ass. *12:* 526 (1975).

17 Winchester, J.F.: Clinical application of hemoperfusion in uremia; in Artificial organs, p. 280 (Macmillan, London 1977).

18 Gelfand, M.C.; Knepshield, J.H.; Cohan, S.; Ramirez, B.; Schreiner, G.E.: Treatment of hepatic coma with hemoperfusion through polyacrylamide hydrogel coated charcoal. Kidney int. *10:* 5239 (1976).

19 Gelfand, M.C.: Charcoal hemoperfusion in treatment of drug overdosage. Dialysis Transplant. *6:* 8 (1977).

20 Gelfand, M.C.; Winchester, J.F.: Hemoperfusion results in uremia. Clin. Nephrol. *11:* 107 (1979).
21 Gutman, R.A.; Stead, W.W.; Robinson, R.R.: Physical activity and employment status of patients on maintenance dialysis. New Engl. J. Med. *6:* 309 (1981).
22 Henderson, L.W.; Colton, C.K.; Ford, C.: Kinetics of hemodiafiltration. Clinical characterization of a new blood cleansing modality. J. Lab. clin. Med. *85:* 372 (1975).
23 Klinkmann, H.; Falkenhagen, D.; Courtney, J.M.: Blood purification by hemoperfusion. Int. J. artif. Organs *2:* 296 (1979).
24 Oreopulos, D.G.: Continuous ambulatory peritoneal dialysis in Canada. Can. med. Ass. J. *6:* 120 (1979).

S. Stefoni, MD, Nephrology and Dialysis Department, St. Orsola University Hospital, Via Massarenti 9, I–40138 Bologna (Italy)

Contr. Nephrol., vol. 29, pp. 133–142 (Karger, Basel 1982)

Multicentric Experience with Combined Hemodialysis/Hemoperfusion in Chronic Uremia

V. Bonomini[a,1], *S. Stefoni*[a,1], *C.U. Casciani*[b,2], *M. Taccone Gallucci*[b,2], *A. Albertazzi*[c], *P. Cappelli*[c], *V. Mioli*[d], *R. Boggi*[d], *F. Mastrangelo*[e], *S. Rizzelli*[e]

[a] Institute of Nephrology and Dialysis, University of Bologna, Italy;
[b] Institute of Surgical Pathology, University of Rome, Italy;
[c] Department of Nephrology and Dialysis, University of Chieti, Italy;
[d] Department of Nephrology and Dialysis, University of Ancona, Italy;
[e] Department of Nephrology and Dialysis, Lecce, Italy

Introduction

The use of charcoal hemoperfusion in the treatment of chronic renal failure has been proposed and applied by several authors [1, 2, 4, 5, 9] while the availability of coating membranes of increased biocompatibility [3] currently allows a safer and wider use of this purifying technique.

It has been recently demonstrated [6, 7] that a long-term treatment of combined hemodialysis/hemoperfusion (HD/HP) yields an improvement of certain dialysis-resistant uremic signs in patients on regular dialysis treatment (RDT), while in selected patients it affords a marked reduction (up to one-third) in the overall time of treatment per week. The tolerance of long-term treatment was reported to be good [6].

In line with these findings, a multicentric study has been carried out with two main aims: (1) to see if long-term treatment with charcoal hemoperfusion is really safe and substantially free from side effects; (2) to verify in a larger and more varied population of patients if such long-term treatment actually improves certain uremic signs persisting despite adequate dialysis treatment.

A third phase of this multicentric study (reducing the weekly time of treatment) is currently being worked on.

[1] Supported by CNR grant No. 80.00388.04.
[2] Supported by 'Gruppo nazionale per le gravi insufficienze d'organo'.

Table I. Effects of combined HD/HP treatment on dialysis-resistant clinical signs

Symptoms	Rome	Chieti	Ancona	Lecce	Bologna
Pruritus	++++	no effect	–	–	++++
Asthenia	–	+++	++++	+++	+++
Cramp	–	+++	no effect	–	no effect
Nausea	++	+++	++	++	++
Anorexia	+++	+++	++++	++++	+++
Peripheral neuropathy	+++	++	–	–	+++
Anemia	–	no effect	no effect	no effect	no effect
General status	+++	++++	+++	+++	++++
Pericarditis	–	–	–	–	+++
Osteodystrophy	++	–	–	++	–

Methods

The basic element of the study was the combined HD/HP treatment. As part of this procedure [6] a carbon cartridge is inserted in the dialysis circuit in series with the dialyzer (hollow fiber or flat plate). The cartridge contains 150 g of activated charcoal coated with a highly biocompatible methacrylate-based membrane [8]. It is left in situ throughout the treatment period. Detailed information has been given elsewhere [6] concerning (1) methodology of the combined HD/HP; (2) tolerance; (3) efficacy and effects on clinical, hematochemical and instrumental parameters.

In this multicentric HD/HP study, one combined HD/HP procedure regularly substituted one of the weekly hemodialysis procedures. Five nephrology and dialysis departments took part in the study: in Bologna, Rome, Chieti, Ancona and Lecce.

Patients and Results

Bologna

Characteristics and results of the 13 Bologna patients have been reported in detail elsewhere [6].

Rome

8 patients (mean age 42) were treated with the HD/HP program for 12 weeks. They had been on RDT from 11 to 118 months, with three dialyses per week (mean 13.9 h). Despite technically adequate treatment, patients complained of pruritus (6/8), nausea and inappetence (5/8), severe peripheral neuropathy (4/8) and severe osteodystrophy (2/8). All patients were generally not feeling healthy.

Table I reports the effects of the HD/HP treatment on the above-mentioned dialysis-resistant symptoms.

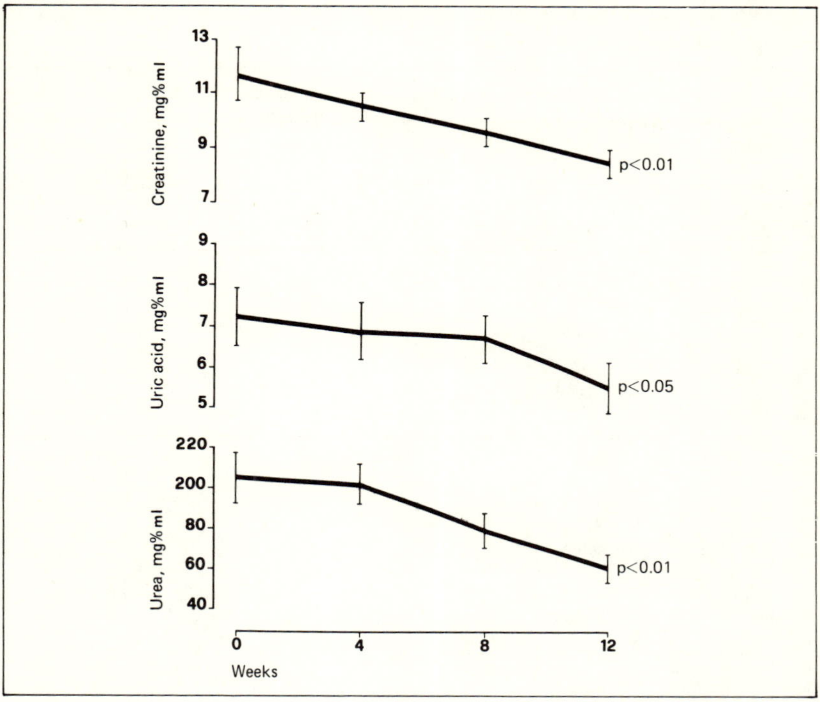

Fig. 1. Effects of HD/HP treatment on plasma values of creatinine, uric acid and urea. Patients from Rome.

Figure 1 shows the changes in plasma creatinine, uric acid and urea levels with time. The decrease in plasma levels during HD/HP is statistically significant (table II).

Figure 2 shows the effects of one single HD/HP procedure on white blood cells. Leucopenia, with lymphocytosis, reached a maximum after 30 min of treatment and is similar to that occurring in standard dialysis procedures with cuprophan membrane.

In 2 patients, the treatment was interrupted after 4 and 6 weeks, respectively, owing to the onset of hypotension during the combined HD/HP procedure. There was no change in platelets, fibrinogen and white and red cells. During a total number of 96 combined HD/HP procedures there occurred 6 incidents of hypotension, 2 chills, and 3 cases of cutaneous rash at the beginning of the procedure. This last side effect, which rapidly disappeared without therapy, was no longer found after a more appropriate dilution of heparin in the cartridge washing fluid (1,500 ml).

Table II. Percentage decrease of plasma values of creatinine, uric acid and urea after 3 months of combined HD/HP treatment

	Rome	Chieti	Ancona	Lecce	Bologna
Creatinine	−27.3	−9.9	+4.6	−2.6	−14.8
Uric Acid	−23.6	−17.2	−17.0	−15.2	−25.6
Urea	−21.9	−11.0	−20.0	−9.7	−19.2

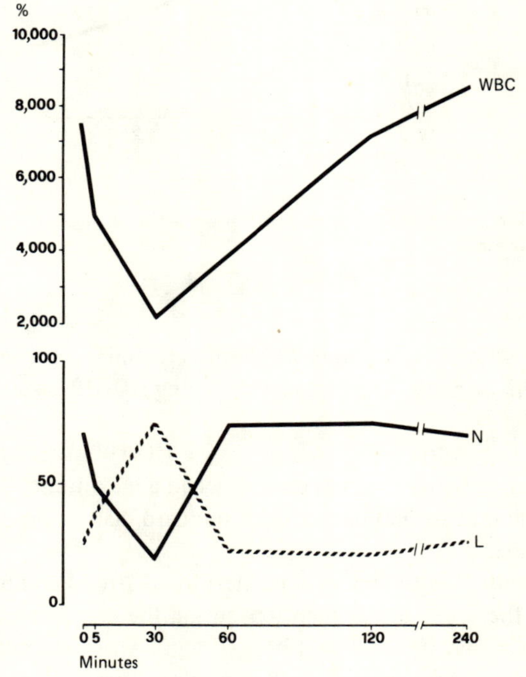

Fig. 2. Effects of a single HD/HP procedure on total white cells (WBC), neutrophils (N) and lymphocytes (L).

Table III. Plasma values (mg%ml) of creatinine, uric acid and urea before and after HD/HP treatment (patients from Chieti)

	Before treatment	After treatment
Creatinine	12.10 ± 2.88	10.90 ± 3.59
Uric acid	5.33 ± 1.85	4.46 ± 1.54
Urea	169.40 ± 56.09	150.87 ± 48.92

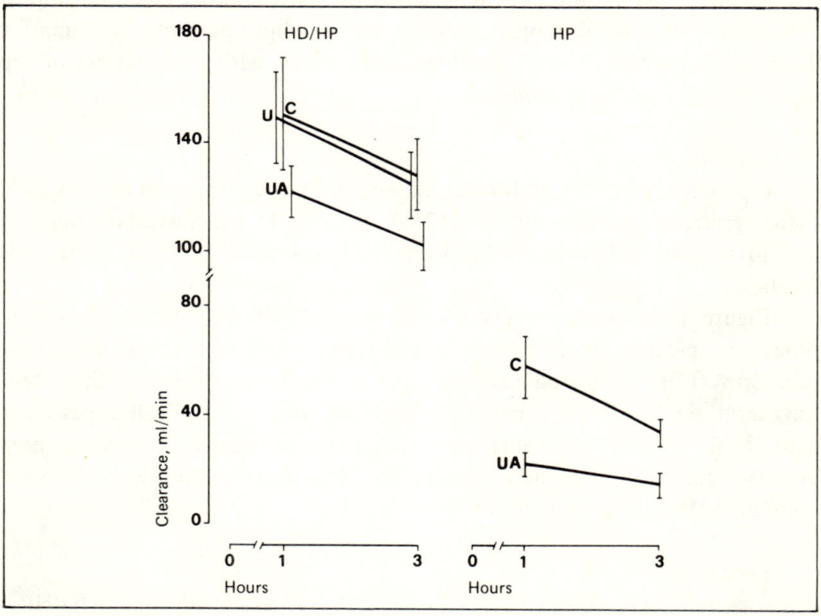

Fig. 3. Clearance of creatinine (C), uric acid (UA) and urea (U) for cartridge plus dialyzer (HD/HP) and cartridge alone (HP) after 1 and 3 h from the beginning of treatment.

Chieti

6 patients (3 males, 3 females) aged 20–53 years, which had been on RDT for 4–60 months were treated with the combined HD/HP program for up to 20 weeks. All patients were on three dialyses per week (12–15 h). They complained of anemia (2/6), pruritus (1/6), asthenia (5/6), and cramp (1/6). 1 patient was treated for 5 weeks, 1 for 12, 1 for 13 and 3 for up to 20 weeks. Table III shows the mean values of creatinine, uric acid and urea before and after treatment. The percentage decrease of these values is reported in table II.

Figure 3 shows the creatinine and uric acid clearance values both for the overall HD/HP system and for the 150-g charcoal cartridge alone, after 1 and 3 h of treatment. Motor nerve conduction velocity (MNCV), which was lower than normal in 4 patients (40.12 ± 8.80 m/s), slightly increased after the combined treatment (41.96 ± 1.57 m/s). Anemia proved unaffected in the 2 severely anemic patients.

As for clinical signs (table I), no effect was achieved in the patient suffering from pruritus. The treatment was stopped at the patient's request after 5 weeks. Cramp disappeared completely after 3 weeks of treatment. 5 patients showed a significant improvement of their well-being.

Hypotension during HD/HP procedures was the most common unpleasant side effect. Plasma fibrinogen, electrolytes and lipid patterns were unaffected. There were two episodes of clotting of the circuit with usual dosage of heparin and standard washing procedure.

Ancona

6 patients were treated for 12–16 weeks. They complained of severe anemia (4/6), gastrointestinal symptoms (2/6), asthenia (5/6), muscular cramp (1/6), and of lack of well-being (5/6). Table I summarizes the effects of the HD/HP treatment.

Figure 4 shows the effects of combined HD/HP on plasma values of creatinine, uric acid and urea. Creatinine was unaffected, while uric acid and, above all, urea ($p < 0.01$) decreased markedly (table II). Table IV shows the effects of long-term treatment on hematocrit, platelets, red cells and all types of white cells. Table V shows the values of plasma renin activity. The most common side effects were chills, headache, fever, vomiting and hypotension. However, no combined HD/HP session had to be interrupted.

Lecce

6 patients were treated for 12–20 weeks. The indications for HD/HP treatment were severe anemia (3/6), severe hyperparathyroidism (4/6), asthenia (2/6), and gastrointestinal symptoms (2/6).

Table VI shows the mean values of plasma creatinine, uric and urea before and after treatment. Creatinine remained unchanged while uric acid and urea (table II) decreased.

Lipids, white cells, platelets and fibrinogen were unaffected. MNCV, which was in the normal range at the beginning of treatment, remained unchanged (51.0 m/s ± 7.7 versus 50.7 ± 3.8).

As for clinical signs, the most positive effects were on general state and inappetence (table I). The treatment had no beneficial effect on severely anemic patients.

Plasma values of PTH were found to decrease. A complete analysis of the effect of the HD/HP treatment on the acid-base balance is undergoing evaluation.

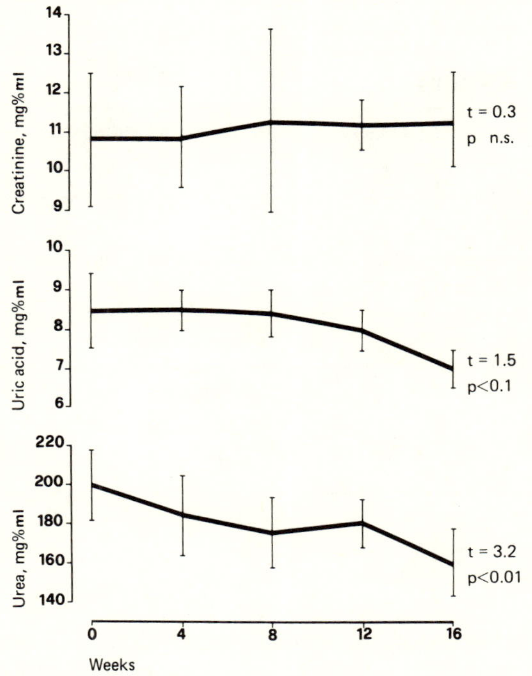

Fig. 4. Effects of HD/HP treatment on plasma values of creatinine, uric acid and urea. Patients from Ancona.

Table IV. Effects of combined HD/HP treatment on Hct, red cells (RBC) and white cells (WBC)

	Basal	4 weeks	8 weeks	12 weeks	16 weeks
RBC, n/mm³ × 1,000	2,222 ± 6,38	2,218 ± 500	2,180 ± 430	2,200 ± 457	2,214 ± 292
WBC, n/mm³	5,080 ± 1,790	5,300 ± 1,500	5,200 ± 1,345	5,400 ± 1,440	5,000 ± 1,570
Neutrophils, %	67.80 ± 5.22	62.30 ± 6.10	60.00 ± 4.33	62.23 ± 5.21	59.40 ± 8.76
Eosinophils, %	2.00 ± 1.22	2.01 ± 1.15	2.00 ± 1.16	2.48 ± 1.14	2.60 ± 1.14
Basophils, %	–	–	–	–	–
Lymphocytes, %	27.40 ± 5.68	28.28 ± 4.67	30.03 ± 5.27	31.23 ± 6.34	36.00 ± 9.00
Monocytes, %	2.60 ± 1.15	2.50 ± 1.17	2.48 ± 1.19	2.53 ± 0.88	2.40 ± 0.55
Platelets, n/mm³ × 1,000	131 ± 33	130 ± 30	133 ± 28	134 ± 27	137 ± 27
Hct, %	19.2 ± 5.26	19.01 ± 4.23	19.00 ± 3.67	20.34 ± 3.33	21.00 ± 2.00

Table V. Effects of HD/HP treatment on plasma renin activity (PRA)

	PRA, ng/ml/h		
	Basal	2 months	4 months
Lying	4.61 ± 0.93	3.85 ± 0.53	4.50 ± 1.00
Standing	6.74 ± 1.23	5.78 ± 0.94	6.72 ± 1.34

Table VI. Plasma values (mg%ml) of creatinine, uric acid and urea before and after HD/HP treatment (patients from Lecce)

	Before treatment	After treatment
Creatinine	10.98 ± 0.87	10.68 ± 1.7
Uric acid	4.56 ± 1.18	3.8 ± 0.46
Urea	1.86 ± 0.43	1.68 ± 0.38

Discussion

Despite the difficulty of following exactly the same protocol in the treatment of RDT patients, both the treated patients and the treatment itself can be taken as homogeneous enough. The results of this multicentric experience give rise to some reflections on the biocompatibility, tolerance, and clinical, hematochemical and metabolic effects of long-term uses of combined HD/HP treatment in chronic uremic patients.

Tolerance and Biocompatibility

The biocompatibility of long-term treatment using charcoal coated with the methacrylate-based membrane has been confirmed as satisfactory. No effect was documented in any patient on red and white cells, platelets, fibrinogen or other hematochemical parameters. As for tolerance, it can be said that the most important side effect is hypotension which generally takes place in severely anemic patients. Most probably, hypovolemia plays a decisive role.

Effects on Clinical Signs

This study confirms the efficacy of the HD/HP treatment concerning the patients' general state, asthenia, nausea, anorexia, well-being, and peripheral neuropathy. MNCV increased in those patients in whom it was lower than normal. This increase is always accompanied by an improvement in clinical signs of peripheral neuropathy. None of the patients treated had pericarditis; it was not possible, therefore, to check the efficacy of HD/HP treatment on this uremic sign [6].

The treatment had little or no effect on muscular cramp.

Hematochemical and Metabolic Effects

All investigators (5/5) confirmed a marked decrease (mean −16.3%) in plasma urea and uric acid (mean −19.7%) values after several weeks of treatment, while 3 of 5 investigators also found a decrease in plasma creatinine (table II). Changes in the generation rate of some metabolites undoubtedly occur during the combined HD/HP treatment. This point of undeniable interest requires further investigation especially in regard to the nitrogen balance and hormonal patterns of the patients. These results clearly show that the HD/HP treatment has no beneficial effect on anemia. This observation, together with the fact that hypotension is more frequent in patients with severe anemia, makes it inadvisable to perform the HD/HP program in severely anemic patients, even though red blood cells per se are unaffected.

Preliminary data on osteodystrophy and PTH levels require further investigation. No effect was found on calcium, phosphate, sodium, potassium, plasma osmolarity or other routine parameters.

In conclusion, it can be said that long-term HD/HP treatment has been confirmed by this multicentric experience as an effective and risk-free therapeutic procedure. As for its efficacy, an exact knowledge of the scope and limits of the charcoal sorption capacity and the most careful selection of patients according to their clinical and metabolic conditions, are indispensable for an appropriate and rational use of combined HD/HP programs.

Summary

A multicentric study was carried out to investigate the safety and effectiveness of long-term treatment of chronic uremic patients by a regular combination of hemodialysis and charcoal hemoperfusion. 39 RDT patients from five dialysis centers were treated for up to 12 months. The combined treatment proved to be safe, well tolerated and effective in improving certain dialysis-resistant uremic signs, mainly severe peripheral neuropathy, asthenia, anorexia, nausea, lack of well-being and relapsing pericarditis. There was also a marked decrease, after several weeks of combined treatment, in plasma values of urea, uric acid and creatinine.

References

1 Chang, T.M.S.: Hemoperfusion alone and in series with ultrafiltration or dialysis for uremia, poisoning and liver failure. Kidney Int. *10:* 305 (1976).

2 Chang, T.M.S.: Assessments of clinical trials of charcoal hemoperfusion in uremic patients. Clin. Nephrol. *11:* 111 (1979).

3 Chang, T.M.S.: Hemoperfusion in 1981 (this issue).

4 Gelfand, M.C.; Winchester, J.F.: Hemoperfusion results in uremia. Clin. Nephrol. *11:* 107 (1979).

5 Klinkmann, H.; Falkenhagen, D.; Courtney, J.M.: Blood purification by hemoperfusion, Int. J. artif. Organs *2:* 296 (1979).

6 Stefoni, S.; Coli, L.; Feliciangeli, G.; Baldrati, L.; Bonomini, V.: Regular hemoperfusion in regular dialysis treatment. A long-term study. Int. J. artif. Organs *3:* 348 (1980).

7 Stefoni, S.; Colì, L.; Feliciangeli, G.; Bonomini, V.: Combined hemodialysis/hemoperfusion treatment as a mean to reduce the weekly hours of treatment in RDT patients, Int. J. artif. Organs *4:* 186 (1981)

8 Stefoni, S.; Feliciangeli, G.; Colì, L.; Bonomini, V.: Evaluation of a new coated charcoal for hemoperfusion in uremia. Int. J. artif. Organs *2:* 320 (1979).

9 Winchester, J.F.: Clinical application of hemoperfusion in uremia; in: Artificial organs, p. 280 (Macmillan Press, London 1977).

V. Bonomini, MD, Nephrology and Dialysis Department,
St. Orsola University Hospital, I–40100 Bologna (Italy)

Contr. Nephrol., vol. 29, pp. 143–148 (Karger, Basel 1982)

Postheparin Lipolytic Activity in Uremic Patients Treated by Hemofiltration[1]

S. Di Giulio, B. Lacour, N.K. Man, F. Martinez-Natera, P. Faguer, T. Drüeke, J.L. Funck-Brentano[2]

Inserm. U 90, Département de Néphrologie, Hôpital Necker, Paris, France

Introduction

Plasma triglyceride concentration is often increased in uremic patients; this lipid anomaly associated with a decrease in high density lipoprotein (HDL) cholesterol may account for the accelerated atherosclerosis observed in patients with chronic renal failure and it can lead to ischemic events [3, 16, 19]. Hypertriglyceridemia may result either from increased synthesis or from decreased catabolism of triglycerides or both. The decreased catabolism of the triglyceride-rich very low density (VLDL) lipoproteins in hemodialysis patients appears to be related to several factors such as carnitine deficiency [2, 12] and impaired lipolytic activity [7, 11]. The activity of the lipoprotein lipase, the main enzyme involved in triglyceride clearance, is generally reduced in uremic patients when measured directly on adipose tissue or indirectly by plasma postheparin lipolytic activity (PHLA) [1, 10, 11]. This reduction seems to be associated with the inhibition of lipoprotein lipase by solutes of middle or high molecular weight [5]: uremic serum inhibits the lipoprotein lipase extracted from normal adipose tissue and activated by normal serum [1]. In vitro dialysis blunts this inhibition [15] and hemofiltration can actually improve PHLA from patients with end-stage renal failure starting a replacement treatment by artificial kidney [7, 9, 14, 20].

The aim of the present work was (1) to study the effect of hemofiltration on the lipid anomalies of uremic patients already treated by intermittent hemodialysis; (2) to compare the effect of one hemofiltration session with that of one

[1] This work was partly supported by the Fondation Simone et Cino del Duca.

[2] We gratefully acknowledge the secretarial work of Mrs. *B. Déruti-Windsor.*

hemodialysis session on PHLA of uremic patients and (3) to investigate whether a fraction of uremic plasma was possibly responsible for the observed inhibition of the lipolytic functions.

Patients and Methods

Plasma PHLA in Patients with End-Stage Renal Failure

PHLA was measured according to the method of *Fredrickson* et al. [8] in healthy control subjects after a 12-hour fast (n = 10) and in patients with chronic renal failure (n = 14) at the first session of a regular hemodialysis treatment (creatinine clearance ⩽5 ml/min). A dose of 0.1 mg/kg body weight (BW) heparin was administered as an intravenous bolus injection. Plasma samples were collected 10 min after heparin administration. The lipolytic activity was then determined using Intralipid® (Vitrum, Sweden) as substrate. Results are expressed as nanomoles of free fatty acids liberated per minute and per milliliter of plasma.

Plasma PHLA in Uremic Patients with Hypertriglyceridemia: Comparison between One Hemofiltration and One Hemodialysis Session

PHLA was measured in uremic patients (n = 3) with hypertriglyceridemia (⩾2.0 mmol/l) after a 12-hour fast. The test was performed the day after the hemofiltration or the hemodialysis session in patients already on intermittent hemodialysis treatment (⩾6 months). A dose of 1 mg/kg BW of heparin was administered as an intravenous bolus injection. One hemofiltration session was performed by a postdilution system of 20 liters using an RP6 (Rhône-Poulenc) artificial kidney equipped with AN 69 1-m^2 polyacrilonitrile membrane [17, 18]. The substitution fluid contained (in mmol/l): sodium 145, potassium 1.0, calcium 1.75, chloride 106, acetate 40 and magnesium 1.7; it was glucose-free. Intermittent hemodialysis treatment consisted of 4-hour sessions thrice weekly on a 1-m^2 plate dialyzer equipped with cuprophane. Dialysate composition was the same as that of the substitution fluid in hemofiltration and it was delivered by a 75-liter dialysate closed batch system (Rhodial 75). An intravenous fat tolerance test [4] was performed 4 h after the end of each session: 1 ml/kg BW Intralipid® 20% was infused into the arteriovenous fistula; then a bolus of 1 mg/kg heparin was injected, plasma samples were collected every 10 min during 1 h. The samples were processed by nephelometry (OD 600 nm) and Intralipid® clearance rate was calculated by a computer as the slope of disappearance of turbidity ($\log_{10}$OD 600 nm) as a function of time (min). Results were expressed as means ± SEM. Peak b_{4-2} was measured in plasma as a marker of middle molecular weight substances before and after either session according to the procedure of *Man* and *Funck-Brentano* [6, 13].

Table I. PHLA (free fatty acids, nmol/ml · min) after hemodialysis and homofiltration

Patient	Hemodialysis	Hemofiltration
1	85.55	126.83
2	73.33	97.99
3	129.99	210.99
Mean	96.29	145.27
SEM	17.21	33.89

Table II. Plasma concentration before (C_0) and after (C_t) hemodialysis and hemofiltration

Patient	Solute	Hemodialysis		Hemofiltration	
		C_0	C_t	C_0	C_t
1	urea, mmol/l	26.6	13.3	24.6	13.2
	creatinine, μmol/l	1,061	601	973	549
	b_{4-2}, mg/l	2.9	1.2	2.9	0.8
2	urea, mmol/l	36.6	18.3	31.0	19.0
	creatinine, μmol/l	1,283	779	1,239	770
	b_{4-2}, mg/l	6.4	2.7	5.4	1.8
3	urea, mmol/l	24.0	15.0	27.0	18.0
	creatinine, μmol/l	1,070	743	1,106	743
	b_{4-2}, mg/l	3.2	1.3	3.1	1.0

Results

PHLA in Patients with End-Stage Renal Failure

Mean PHLA was decreased in end-stage renal failure patients when compared to that of control subjects : 22.9 ± 4.8 (SEM) versus 78.5 ± 9.8 nmol/ml · min ($p < 0.001$).

PHLA in Patients with Hypertriglyceridemia: Comparison between Hemofiltration and Hemodialysis

Mean plasma PHLA was higher after a hemofiltration session than after a hemodialysis session (table I) : 145.2 ± 33.8 (SEM) after hemofiltration and 96.2 ± 17.2 nmol/ml · min after hemodialysis. Mean Intralipid® clearance rate was higher after hemofiltration when compared to hemodialysis: 0.0123 ± 0.003 (SEM) after hemofiltration and 0.0104 ± 0.001 after hemodialysis. Table II shows the individual values of plasma urea, creatinine and peak b_{4-2} concentra-

Table III. Removal rate $\frac{C_0 - C_t}{C_0}$ per session (%) in hemodialysis and hemofiltration

Patient	Solute	Hemodialysis	Hemofiltration
1	urea	50	47
	creatinine	43	43
	b_{4-2}	58	72
2	urea	50	45
	creatinine	39	37
	b_{4-2}	57	66
3	urea	37	33
	creatinine	30	32
	b_{4-2}	59	67

tions in the 3 patients before (C_0) and after (C_t) each session. No significant difference appeared for C_0 before hemodialysis and hemofiltration. Table III shows the individual removal rates of urea, creatinine and peak b_{4-2} during hemodialysis and hemofiltration.

Figure 1 shows the mean removal rate of urea, creatinine and peak b_{4-2} during hemodialysis and hemofiltration: it was 0.46 ± 0.04 (SEM) for urea, 0.37 ± 0.04 for creatinine, and 0.58 ± 0.02 for peak b_{4-2} in hemodialysis and 0.42 ± 0.04 for urea, 0.37 ± 0.03 for creatinine, and 0.68 ± 0.02 for peak b_{4-2} with hemofiltration. The removal rate was higher for urea with hemodialysis and for peak b_{4-2} with hemofiltration, whereas no difference was observed with either procedure for creatinine.

Discussion

Plasma PHLA is decreased in uremic patients with hypertriglyceridemia. Inhibition of tissue-activated lipoprotein lipase extracts has been suggested to occur from middle [15] or high molecular weight [5] substances. We failed to observe a decrease in plasma PHLA when activated PHLA from control subjects was incubated with plasma ultrafiltrate obtained in vitro from uremic patients without hyperlipidemia [7]. Moreover ultrafiltrates obtained in vivo from the 3 hypertriglyceridemic patients using a highly permeable membrane failed to decrease the plasma PHLA of these uremic patients which improved after one hemofiltration session. Improvement of plasma PHLA in hemodialysis patients even after one hemofiltration session may be related to increased mass transfer of middle or high molecular weight toxins.

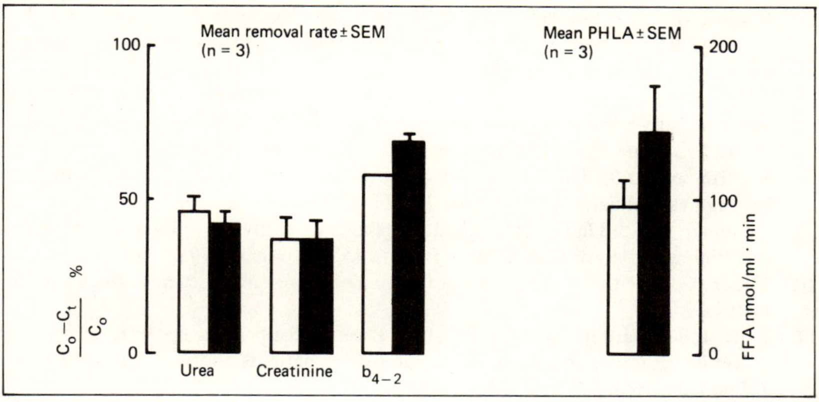

Fig. 1. Mean PHLA and mean removal rates of urea, creatinine and peak b_{4-2} after one hemodialysis session (open columns) and after one hemofiltration session (hatched columns). FFA = Free fatty acids.

Inhibition may involve metabolic steps preceding that of the circulating activated enzymes as detected by PHLA. Investigations using adipose tissue cells incubated with total uremic serum and separated serum fractions are in progress in our laboratory since uremic toxicity may disturb tissue synthesis, secretion or binding to capillary endothelium of lipoprotein lipase.

In conclusion, hemofiltration led to an improvement in plasma PHLA in hemodialysis patients. Further investigations are needed to know whether higher removal rates of middle or high molecular weight substances will be related to a decreased inhibition of lipolytic activities in uremic patients.

References

1 Bagdade, J.D.; Yee, E.; Wilson, D.E.; Shafrir, E.: Hyperlipidemia in renal failure: studies of plasma lipoproteins, hepatic triglyceride production and tissue liproprotein-lipase in chronically uremic rat model. J. Lab. clin. Med. *91:* 176–186 (1978).

2 Bohmer, T.; Bergrem, H.; Eiklid, K.: Carnitine deficiency induced during intermittent hemodialysis for renal failure. Lancet *i:* 126–128 (1978).

3 Brunzell, J.D.: Triglycerides and coronary heart disease. New Engl. J. Med. *303:* 1060 1061 (1980).

4 Chan, M.K.; Varghese, Z.; Persaud, J.W.; Baillod, R.A.; Moorhead, J.F.: Fat clearance before and after heparin in chronic renal failure: hemodialysis reduces post-heparin fractional clearance of intralipid. Clinica chim. Acta. *108:* 95–101 (1980).

5 Crawford, G.A.; Savdie, E.; Stewart, J.H.; Mahony, J.F.: Inhibition of normal plasma lipases by serum from chronic renal failure patients. Trans. Am. Soc. artif. internal Organs. *25:* 426–429 (1979).

6 Cueille, G.: Mise en évidence et évaluation des 'Moyennes molécules' de taille de la vitamine B 12 présentes dans les liquides biologiques des sujets normaux et des patients urémiques. J. Chromatogr., biomed. Appl. *146:* 55–59 (1978).

7 Di Giulio, S.; Lacour, B.; Thevenin, M.; Basile, C.; Drüeke, T.; Man, N.K.: Improvement of post-heparin lipolytic activity (PHLA) after haemofiltration in uraemic patients. Proc. Eur. Dialysis Transplant. Ass. *17:* 259–265 (1980).

8 Fredrickson, D.S.; Ono, K.; Davis, L.L.: Lipolytic activity of post-heparin plasma in hyperglyceridemia. J. Lipid Res. *4:* 24–28 (1963).

9 Henning, H.V.; Balusek, E.: Lipid metabolism in uremic: effect of regular hemofiltration and dialysis treatment. J. Dialysis *1:* 595–606 (1977).

10 Heuck, C.C.; Ritz, E.: Hyperlipoproteinemia in renal insufficiency. Nephron *25:* 1–7 (1980).

11 Ibels, L.S.; Reardon, M.F.; Nestel, P.J.: Plasma post-heparin lipolytic activity and triglyceride clearance in uremic and hemodialysis patients and renal allograft recipients. J. Lab. clin. Med. *87:* 648–659 (1976).

12 Lacour, B.; Di Giulio, S.; Chanard, J.; Ciancioni, C.; Haguet, M.; Lebkiri, B.; Basile, C.; Drüeke, T.; Assan, R.; Funck-Brentano, J.L.: Carnitine improves lipid anomalies in haemodialysis patients. Lancet *ii:* 763–765 (1980).

13 Man, N.K.; Cueille, G.; Zingraff, J.; Boudet, J.; Sausse, A.; Funck-Brentano, J.L.: Uremic neurotoxin in the middle molecular weight range. Artif. Organs *4:* 116–120 (1980).

14 Minear, A.; Minami, E.; Blankenship, J.; Shankel, S.: Lipoprotein-lipase inhibitor removal during hemofiltration of renal failure patients. Abstr. Am. Soc. Nephrol. 47 A (1980).

15 Murase, T.; Cattran, D.C.; Rubstein, B.; Steiner, G.: Inhibition of lipoprotein-lipase by uremic plasma: a possible cause of hypertriglyceridemia. Metabolism *245:* 1279–1286 (1975).

16 Nikkilä, E.A.; Taskinen, M.R.; Kekki, M.: Relation of plasma high density liproprotein cholesterol to liproprotein-lipase activity in adipose tissue and skeletal muscle of man. Atherosclerosis *29:* 497–501 (1978).

17 Quellhorst, E.; Rieger, J.; Doht, B.; Beckmann, H.; Jacob, J.; Kraft, B.; Mietzsch, G.; Scheler, F.: Treatment of chronic uraemia by an ultrafiltration kidney. First clinical experience. Proc. Eur. Dialysis Transplant. Ass. *13:* 314–321 (1976).

18 Quellhorst, E.; Doht, B.; Shuenemann, B.: Hemofiltration: treatment of renal failure by ultrafiltration and substitution. J. Dialysis *1:* 529–544 (1977).

19 Rostand, S.G.; Gretes, J.C.; Kirk, A.K.; Rutsky, E.A.; Andreoli, T.E.: Ischemic heart disease in patients with uremia undergoing maintenance hemodialysis. Kidney int. *16:* 600–611 (1979).

20 Sanfelippo, M.; Grundy, S.; Henderson, L.: Transport of very low density lipoprotein triglyceride: comparison of hemodialysis and hemofiltration (Abstract). Trans. Am. Soc. artif. Internal Organs 868 (1980).

S. Di Giulio, MD, Département de Néphrologie, Hôpital Necker,
161 rue de Sévres, F–75730 Paris Cédex 15 (France)

Subject Index